# WORKING
# OUT,
# WORKING
# WITHIN

The Tao of
Inner Fitness
Through Sports
and Exercise

# WORKING
# OUT,
# WORKING
# WITHIN

JERRY LYNCH, PH.D., AND
CHUNGLIANG AL HUANG

Jeremy P. Tarcher/Putnam
a member of Penguin Putnam Inc.
New York

Most Tarcher/Putnam books are available at special quantity
discounts for bulk purchases for sales promotions, premiums,
fund-raising, and educational needs. Special books or book
excerpts also can be created to fit specific needs. For details,
write or telephone Putnam Special Markets, 200 Madison
Avenue, New York, NY 10016; (212) 951-8891.

Jeremy P. Tarcher/Putnam
a member of
Penguin Putnam Inc.
200 Madison Avenue
New York, NY 10016
www.penguinputnam.com

Library of Congress Cataloging-in-Publication Data

Lynch, Jerry, date.
  Working out, working within : the Tao of inner fitness through
sports and exercise / by Jerry Lynch and Chungliang Al Huang.
      p.   cm.
  "A Jeremy P. Tarcher/Putnam book"—T.p. verso.
  ISBN 0-87477-913-8
  1. Sports—Psychological aspects.  2. Exercise—Psychological aspects.  3. Taoism.  I. Huang, Chungliang Al.  II. Title.
GV 706.4.L96    1997              97-36671 CIP
796'.01—dc21

Book design by Mauna Eichner
Brush calligraphic art by Chungliang Al Huang

Printed in the United States of America
10  9  8  7  6  5  4  3  2  1

This book is printed on acid-free paper. ∞

H-98

*This book
is dedicated to
the natural athlete
in each of us.*

*To Jeremy Tarcher,*
*a man with vision and integrity,*
*our heartfelt appreciation.*

# Contents

# Introduction

Upon winning the twenty-first New York City Marathon, Douglas Wakiihuri of Kenya would say how very relaxed he was as he floated effortlessly over the course with dominating ease. With Zen simplicity, he talked about the marathon as sacred ground, ripe with the fruits of life's truths. When sports journalists asked him about the mundane aspects of mileage, fitness level, racing strategy and diet, he quickly pointed out how such a journey deserves better; there's so much more that this race offers each of us.

All of sport and exercise deserve better. Traditionally, athletics and fitness are battlegrounds for war against an opponent, a clock, scoring goals and other external concerns. The Tao of Inner Fitness, on the other hand, views sports as an arena for the battles within, where your obedience to athletics and fitness cannot be separated from the search for life's verities; the physical life gives our spiritual path a boost as we stare in the face our inner concerns of fear, fatigue, failure, patience, perseverance, courage, confidence, ego, self-doubt and a host of others that affect our growth as athletes and people. What we notice is the way that sport and exercise can transport us to a new level of awareness beyond the game itself, to a place where all of our external successes and accomplishments are the mere reflections of the victories within against these demons.

We not only have the opportunity to become better athletes, we can become better people as well. There's a bittersweet story about a pro football player who is severely injured during a championship game. A woman watching the game on television leans over to her husband as the athlete is carried off the field and says, "I hope this accident makes him a better person." Indeed, we often become better people from athletic adversity. For example, you will see how injury in sports is an opportunity for inner growth, giving you the chance to take time out and reflect and appreciate what you do have. Remember that in Chinese, the word for crisis means both danger and opportunity.

Where the traditional goals of sport and fitness provide much satisfaction and fulfillment, many are realizing that external rewards tend to be unidimensional; we seem to be sensing that there is something much wider and deeper to experience, something that could also enable us to sustain much more enthusiasm and joy for our physical efforts.

The Tao of Inner Fitness is a new, refreshing approach that sees our physical activity as a way to restore total oneness with ourselves and create harmony among body, mind and spirit; under this notion, exercise becomes the means to experiencing a personal potential greater than the physical skills themselves. We (Jerry and Chungliang) notice this need to integrate body, mind and spirit into daily life from our extensive global work with athletes, performers and fitness enthusiasts who see our first book together, *Thinking Body, Dancing Mind,* as a support for this kind of thinking. They tell us that their enjoyment in sport and exercise is directly related to this alignment of body, mind and spirit, a state that the

Japanese refer to as "Satori." These seminarians express a strong desire in taking sports and fitness to this level, to a higher dimension of both physical enjoyment and personal growth. They teach us that they search for greater joy with their physical lives and deeper personal awareness, the celebration of being fully alive, healthy and well; they allude to not only a physical revolution taking place, but a spiritual revolution as well, one that offers a deep, soulful connection to life through the physical experience. Up until now, this spiritual revolution has been kept very separate from its physical counterpart. We seem excited and ready to integrate our physical workouts with the working within of our minds and souls in order to triumph in the biggest game ever, the game of life.

People are now beginning to look for ways to restructure their views, attitudes and beliefs with sports, exercise and fitness. This new shift in consciousness helps you to see sports and exercise as arenas not only for the exploration of your athletic potential and physical growth, but also for accepting the challenges within, where the opponent is yourself and the reward deeply private and personal.

An athlete who has repeatedly demonstrated this new consciousness in sport is pro triathlete Mark Allen, a legendary icon and six-time Hawaiian Ironman champion. In what was his final race before retirement, the "King of Kona" found himself trailing the leader by an almost insurmountable thirteen minutes going into the final stage of the event. The thought of winning was remote and bleak. Yet, he never gave up. The race became a deep, soulful experience for which his challenge was totally within. In what many consider to be the greatest comeback performance in triathlon history, Allen passed Tom Hellriegel three miles from the finish to win his sixth Ironman. According to Allen, it took all he had physically, emotionally and spiritually to make it happen. He talks about how every race teaches you something and you begin to win on a deeper level. Arguably the toughest triathlete ever, Allen touches upon sport as an inner journey when he claims "the race is so real, it's just you against yourself . . . a very pure experience, very enriching." We need to recognize that, like Allen, we are all spiritual beings having a physical experience in which our bodies are temples or homes for our deepest inner selves.

To help us get to that next level, we present this book, *Working Out, Working Within: The Tao of Inner Fitness Through Sports and Exercise*, as a practical, experiential handbook for anyone involved with fitness, exercise, movement and sports who wishes to discover ways to get more out of their physical lives and, also, to help deal with life more effectively. We bring to this book a masterful blend of Eastern philosophy and Western psychology. Lynch, a former national champion, coach and sports psychologist, is an avid student of Tao with a doctorate in psychology. Huang is an expert in the area of Chinese Tao philosophy and master of Tai Ji. Together and throughout this book, we integrate our rich professional backgrounds for the purpose of facilitating both physical and inner fitness, using the ancient teachings and precepts of Tao, combined with principles of sports psychology.

As an example of this new fitness paradigm, consider that when you exercise the body in a way that feels good, you heighten your spirit; when the body is fit, you feel good all over. Here is a book that will help you to create more joy and pleasure while working out and show how you can use sports and fitness activities as powerful catalysts to learn the ancient truths of life—lessons about criticism, patience, mastery, self-reliance, diligence, crisis, loss, loyalty and many others. You can do this because when you are physically stimulated—be it sports, exercise, martial arts, dance or other forms of fitness—pathways to your inner emotional self, as well as to the deep centers of creativity and thought, become opened. In this state of mind and body, you are more receptive to personal growth and change; you are more willing to accept what you now can see as truth, where beforehand, you may have become somewhat defensive and guarded.

*Working Out, Working Within* will also help you to use your sports and physical workouts to become inward bound, away from outer scores and results, and begin to really get to know yourself, test your limits, and discover what you are made of as you become both physically and spiritually fit for the game of life. You will begin to experience inner changes when you learn how to identify your personal rhythms and "work out" to your own inner beat and pace for a higher, more satisfying level of participation.

This book will help you be calm and relaxed during your workout and experience more vitality, energy, fluidity and spontaneity with your physical regimes. You will be able to sustain your workouts more easily as you experience the universal benefit of being internally fit. More fun is in store as you recapture the deeper qualities of excitement, curiosity, wonderment and enthusiasm for sports and exercise.

All of us who partake in sports and physical fitness activities need to go at our own pace. The timing must be right; you need to follow your heart and intuitive sense. When the fruit is ready, it does not need to be talked into falling from the tree. With time, we believe that most of us will seek ways to sustain our physical programs and search for inner fulfillment as well as we take it to the next level. It is a process that refuses to yield to demographic boundaries; all ability levels and ages are invited to take the journey regardless of your sport or physical activity of choice. In this sense, this book is written for all who (or would like to) engage in regular physical activity, whether a professional or collegiate athlete, national champion, Olympian, dancer, martial artist, weekend warrior, fitness fanatic or neophyte (one who wishes to begin a lifestyle of total fitness). We have designed it also for all coaches, trainers, teachers, athletic directors and sports medicine professionals. It will help us all create not only a new frame of mind, but also a refreshing frame of heart for mastering the bigger game of life. After all, sport is a good metaphor for life while life, itself, becomes a sport.

## HOW TO USE THIS BOOK

*Working Out, Working Within* is extremely user-friendly. In the introduction, we set the tone for the paradigm shift, one that will help you to see beyond traditional attitudes toward sports and exercise in which physical activity can be experienced as a tool for personal transformation on the path to inner fitness. Once aligned with this shift in consciousness, you are ready to begin this exciting journey by learning the four basic techniques that will facilitate your movement within. These techniques are the building blocks—the cornerstones—that form the foundation from which you will build your program for working out and working within. It is in the Starting Out section that you are introduced to the ancient Chinese philosophy of Tao, the basis for all attitudinal shifts and cognitive restructuring techniques used throughout your journey. Become very familiar with Part I before you attempt to handle the material that follows. It is a prerequisite for success on the journey of inner fitness.

Once you have a thorough understanding of these basic techniques, you will be ready for Part 2. This section introduces the five stages of inner and outer fitness and shows you how to liberally apply these tools when appropriate. We will guide you at each stage to be sure you don't get sidetracked along the way.

At this juncture, you may be wondering how to progress through the stages: straight through or skip around? There is a logical sequence to the placement of the stages. We believe that it is necessary to hurdle your self-imposed limitations before you can begin the process of physical resurgence. Once you begin to engage in your physical program, you are in a better position to consider that the possibilities for physio-spiritual fitness are, indeed, unlimited. From this position, you are better equipped to go more deeply within and face the more difficult inner demons, such as loss, opponents, ego and letting go of the dire necessity to win. Finally, you are now ready, having experienced the previous four stages, to use your physical life as a meditation, a way to develop stillness in motion and give in to your most creative self. It is here that you put it all together and "walk your talk" in cooperation with the natural rhythms of self and all that surrounds you. We suggest at the outset that you read each in the order of their occurrence as steps along the path. Metaphorically speaking, you wouldn't try to run ten miles until you could handle five.

Once through the sequence of stages, we encourage you to use the book by periodically checking in and randomly selecting those issues or chapters that are of immediate concern to you. In this way, the book becomes a close companion available to meet your needs at a moment's notice. We suggest that you keep it by your bed for reading prior to sleep or in your workout training bag for immediate reference prior to your physical activity. Since you have developed a solid foundation by your initial exposure, you can now be creative and introduce topics in any way you deem appropriate; open the book at random, read the short passage that appears and meditate upon it as you doze off into dreamland or go for your daily walk, run or other type of workout. As you engage in exercise or sport, the reading of a random chapter can serve as the T.O.D. —thought of the day—to guide you inward for spiritual reflections during your sport or workout regime.

Finally, Part 3 serves as a personal metaphor to encourage you to "break out" on your own and discover your own personal body-mind-spirit connection. Perhaps you will want to write your own metaphor to serve as a strong positive touchstone helping you to contact, at will, your personal sense of the physical encounter of the spiritual kind.

# PART 1

# Starting Out

*Techniques for*

*Cultivating*

*Inner Talent*

In this first part of the journey, we want you to focus on cultivating your inherent, natural inclination toward inner fitness. We use the concept "inner talent" because like any talent, it is a gift with which you are naturally endowed, an ability that once nurtured and encouraged, will bloom to its full potential.

To help in this cultivation process, we offer you the following four chapters, which contain the tools and strategies that will help you to experience deeper inner fitness through your physical activity. As with any fitness program, it helps to have the proper equipment and gear. These techniques will make you better equipped by providing the building blocks for each chapter in the five stages of the Tao of Inner Fitness journey.

# Application of
# Ancient Wisdom

## THE PHILOSOPHY OF TAO

Translated more often than any book with the exception of the
Bible, the *Tao Te Ching* (pronounced "dow de jing") has been widely
used as a source of spiritual strength for centuries. By leading you
inward, the Tao helps you to recognize and align with your personal rhythms and pace; by so doing, you bring greater satisfaction,
joy and fulfillment to yourself and your world.

The Chinese calligraphic symbol for Tao is made up of a head
signifying wisdom and a foot representing walking; literally translated it means walking the way of wisdom. This way of wisdom
creates a shift in attitude and consciousness by restructuring your
conceptual view of things. It helps you to see the larger pictures
of nature and blend with them. For example, by shifting your
attitudes, you begin to move beyond failure to opportunity, from
competition to cooperation, from winning as a destination to a
journey.

Even though it is impossible to define the ineffable Tao in
Western terms, by now the concept of Tao has become universally
accepted and known as a commonsensical way for human beings to

cooperate with the course of nature. Tao means the way of natural truth and encourages you to notice how nature works and then act accordingly. Lao Tzu, the mythical sage of ancient China, who is generally acknowledged as the supreme teacher of the Tao, asked that we emulate Tao by using the potent metaphor of the flowing patterns of water in everyday life. Tao is, like water, the path of least resistance. Alan Watts, culminating his brilliant career as the most lucid interpreter of Zen and Tao, chose *Tao: The Watercourse Way* as the title for his last book, thus following in the footsteps of Lao Tzu's teachings.

The twenty-five-hundred-year-old Taoist classic *Tao Te Ching*, with merely 5,000 Chinese words in eighty-one short poetic verses, continues to challenge us with a wide variety of interpretations applicable to the success and fulfillment in all areas of living. In *Working Out, Working Within*, we use the time-honored precepts and teachings of Tao to help you develop your inner fitness through sports and exercise. The following are a few of the most essential concepts of Tao that we will use throughout this book to facilitate the restructuring of the more limited traditional ideas and thought patterns with regard to physical activity:

I. *Tze Jan* (pronounced "dje run"): Spontaneity

Literally, these two Chinese words translate as "Self Naturally So," or being your spontaneous and authentic self. Through sports and exercise, you learn to cultivate personal health and well-being as you delve deeper into self-discovery, who you are and what you are made of in order to grow spiritually. Inner fitness is evident when you recapture the "romance" with the spontaneity of your true nature. With Tao, sports and exercise enable you to look within and become one with your natural self as you learn how to spontaneously transcend your separateness in the unifying vision of body, mind and spirit.

2. *Wu Wei* ("woo way"):  Noninterference

Here is the principle of ultimate cooperative behavior with nature's way, the principle of harmonious action. Wu Wei can be interpreted as an unforced blending with surrounding circumstances without the unnatural imposition of your will. The Tao cyclist works with the wind by drafting behind a team member; the skier refuses to "conquer" the mountain and chooses, instead, to blend with its contours and undulations. You will discover that you gain wisdom by going with the way of nature, instead of opposing it egotistically. When you learn to cooperate with the way things are, instead of insisting on controlling or manipulating situations to your individual wishes, you begin to feel the fluidity and flexibility within your physical activity and the effects of this flow on all arenas of life.

For example, notice what happens to you on a spiritual level when you flow with fatigue and failure rather than fight them. Embrace these demons as necessary adjuncts for the breaking of new ground physically and emotionally. With this line of thought, injury becomes a messenger announcing that change and reflection are in order. Wu Wei is truly the way, the lifestyle of anyone who follows the Tao, the path of least resistance in all that you do.

3. *Tai Ji* ("tie gee"): Stillness in Motion/Movement in Stillness

"Tai" is the centering and expansion of the self. "Ji" is the practice of inner quiescence and focusing while you act and move outwardly in everyday living. With Tai Ji, you learn a new way of being, fully in touch with your inner power as you exercise externally. Tai Ji is a philosophy of living according to the Tao. In sports and in all forms of exercise, you feel the stillness in motion, and you sustain the momentum when you find repose.

4. *Yin Yang:* Polarity Balancing

The Tao teaches that life is composed of balancing opposites, two poles integrated into one concept. Western minds are trained from birth to be dualistic, comfortable amid distinction: you are either in shape or out of shape; either a winner or a loser; too fast or too slow; soft or strong; flexible or inflexible. The Tao makes no split between these polarities; instead it neutralizes them into a whole unity. This paradoxical mystery helps you to develop greater strength, satisfaction and higher levels of participation in sports and exercise.

For example, if you are too Yang, too results- or outcome-oriented, you can become nervous, tense, anxious and stressed. This leads to mistakes, setbacks and possible illness and injury because you refuse to listen to what nature is saying. If you are too Yin, too passive or self-conscious, you can become timid and non-assertive. This can result in being hesitant and unfulfilled, failing to achieve the vast boundaries of your potential.

When you integrate these seemingly conflicting forces, you experience a balancing of the Yin and Yang currents that will keep you aligned and in harmony with the true natural way of sports and exercise. By so doing, you learn to develop the right timing and become more willing to let the "game" come to you, let it evolve at its own pace and tempo. In this consciousness, there is a place for both aggression and passivity, speed and slowing it down. The natural Tao athlete understands this need for balancing and uses it to great advantage.

5. *I Pien* ("yee bee-an"): Change and Transformation

I Pien teaches us to be in tune with the universal rhythm of nature that renews itself in cyclical fashion: we move from day to night, winter to spring; leaves come, leaves go. Ignoring these cycles creates surprising twists that often upset the balance of nature. According to the Tao, everything throughout nature moves along in consistent fashion, always returning to its source. We simply need to notice the cycles and act in harmony with them.

Like nature you have your cycles too. Following them keeps you aligned with Tao. In sports and exercise programs, you become aware of your peaks and ebbs during a single day, a week, month or year in which your energy fluctuates naturally. You learn, according to the Tao, how to play and live more creatively and productively when you accept and adjust to these periods of change.

6. *Yung Qi* ("yu-ing chee"): The Vital Force of Life

Beyond your own breath, Yung Chi is part of your ever-expanding energy life force. Everything around you has Chi, energy you can tap into as you learn to expand what you think are your limits and connect with the outer boundaries of your vast potential. Qi is above and beyond as we reach up to the sky to funnel in the vital force of life; notice how every flower and all foliage turn to the sun and light. There is the Qi of physical as well as atmospheric vibrations in our worldly environment, including our emotional and psychological feelings and the sensing of other human forces around us. And, as above so below, we learn to tap the force of the earth underneath, our feet tapping the vitality of life seeping deep down with our roots.

While you play your sport, workout and exercise, learn to cultivate, conserve and keep your inner and outer Qi flowing. Pay attention to the circulation of Qi inside your body; the Chinese Taoists call this internal meditation the "Circulation of the Golden Light." Focus on the extension and connection of your outgoing Qi to the powerful energy field all around.

7. *Te* ("deh"): Personal Power

Te is the expression of Tao in sports and exercise as well as all of life; in Chinese, Te means personal power. When you develop Te, you are able to fulfill your greatest potential. Te is developed when you see setbacks and failures as strengths, opportunities to learn; when you stop trying and simply dare to "do" your physical life; when you stay in the moment and put aside the outcomes or results; when you cease to be self-critical and merely accept the true natural self; when you exhibit courage and personal integrity at the risk of being different; when you seek the spiritual connection in all that you do and align yourself with the joy and fun of life. And, as is the case with all Chinese paradox, your ultimate Te or power is achieved when you don't seek power at all; the process of seeking is one that will tire you. It is best to take action with enthusiasm and not be overly concerned about what happens.

Te is also the miraculous natural functioning of simply being natural, as in the flowering of plants. In humans, there is the formation of eyes and ears, the circulation of blood, and the reticulation of nerves, which all come about without conscious direction. By tuning inward to the miracle of the human body, with all its natural perfection, we can harness our personal power without effort.

The ideogram of Te means going along with the unity of eye and heart mind (Xing). At its root, Te is personal power exercised without the use of force or undue interference, according to the Tao wisdom of Tze Jan and Wu Wei.

8. *Feng Liu* ("fong lee-you"):  Windflow Grace

Tao is often described as the Watercourse Way, or following the way of the windflow. Contrasting with the self-conscious striving of most people, followers of Tao naturally swim downstream and catch the wind, enjoying the art of sailing, instead of rowing the boat and pushing against the current. The graceful style of a cheerful, easygoing person is admired for the "feng liu" personality.

Combined with the virtue of Te, Feng Liu is another highly esteemed quality to be cultivated, along with spontaneity (Tze Jan), noninterference (Wu Wei), and the flexibility and adaptability to change and transform (I Pien).

As you begin your five-stage journey, you will notice how we weave these Tao precepts and philosophical tenets in subtle ways throughout the lessons for creating the Tao of inner fitness. We strongly encourage you to notice how these universal principles also can be applied to your everyday games of life. Their influence permeates all aspects of your living Tao journey.

In keeping with the theme of Tao, each of the five stages on your journey will be introduced with Chinese calligraphy, a seven-thousand-year-old abstract art form. Considered by some to be the essence of energy (Chi) development, this dance of thought will prepare you to open your heart to the Tao precepts that await you within each chapter.

# Breath Watching

## MEDITATION WITH A TAO MIND

The first technique or skill for cultivating inner talent is breath watching, a simple yet effective method of meditation creating what we call the Tao Mind. Tao Mind, in Chinese, is actually Tao Xing (Hsing), a more inclusive symbol that suggests both heart and mind. According to Tao Xing, there is no separation between the intellect and the feeling heart. Thoughts stem from both the heart and brain.

The Tao Mind is a state of calm, effortless, relaxed, focused meditation, one that ultimately helps you to become one with the ball, the bike, the racquet, the terrain and with yourself in all of life. The Tao Mind is the place from which you can eventually achieve deep insight into what were once blurry issues and concerns; you may obtain clarity about life's direction from this state. It can help you to problem solve, make decisions and even help you to answer life's important questions, such as: Who am I? Where am I going? And with whom?" This Tao Mind is a pathway into your deeper, healthier self.

The Tao Mind also will help you to improve your overall performance and interest in sports and fitness, sustaining and main-taining your enthusiasm and satisfaction in physical activity. Simply put, integrating your body, mind and spirit in this way creates workouts that truly feel good, naturally. Your physical routines will begin to flow more easily, with greater comfort, minimal effort, and less strain. When this happens, you become more apt to con-tinue your physical endeavors for as long as you live.

This Tao Mind meditation is the state of mind from which we will introduce the techniques of visual recording and affirmation reciting. When you do this, all tension is reduced and your body-mind-spirit will be in sync, opening the window of opportunity for spiritual expansion and optimal performance.

Also, the Tao Mind is a natural companion to be used prior to any physical endeavor. It helps you to experience the moment-to-moment process of your sport or exercise. Being in this state opens up the possibility of experiencing "swimming downstream," a state in which the ball looks bigger, or the goal seems enlarged, when it all comes together, when you feel invincible. This state tends to occur when you first enter the Tao Mind for five or ten minutes, then, through visual recording, focus on *what* you do, the process, as opposed to *how* you do, a commentary on the product or results. Too many of us, by focusing on winning, points scored, yards gained and other outcomes, take ourselves completely out of this state of mind.

To help you gain access to the Tao Mind and eventually enter into a more relaxed groove for effortless performance and greater awareness for extended periods of time, we offer you a simple, easy-to-learn technique that will calm, relax and energize you. It is called breath watching.

Most of us take very shallow breaths through our mouths with

considerable amounts of usable oxygen lost in the process of repeated exhalation. A more natural, effective method of respiration
is to breathe through the nostrils and allow the breath to penetrate
and circulate throughout the entire body, from your head down to
your toes. To do this effectively, imagine the incoming air as if it
were a white cloud filled with pure oxygen. Watch this white cloud
enter your nostrils as you slowly breathe in. While elongating your
breath, imagine the pure white air permeating your lungs, entering
the bloodstream and making its way to all parts of the body; slowly
release the residue and see it exit the nostrils as a smoky, de-oxygenated cloud and rise up to the sky dissolving into oblivion.

Notice how deer, horses and most other animals use their
noses to breathe while running. Breathing through your nostrils
and allowing the oxygen to filter through the entire body will help
you to gain quicker access to the Tao Mind in which performance
and inner fitness can be optimized. This approach may seem difficult at first, but once you begin to practice it on a consistent basis,
in time you will grow more adept and find it to be quite natural.
You will eventually, if not immediately, begin to empty the mind in
a state of quiet meditation where you achieve what is called inner
stillness. Ultimately, you will carry this over to your physical activity to create stillness in motion, where body-mind-spirit are in syn-
chronicity.

Try this breath-watching technique while sitting comfortably
in a chair, keeping your back naturally upright, your feet planted in
front, with legs open naturally from your hips, and eyes closed to
reduce external stimulation.

- Inhale slowly through nostrils and watch with your eyes
  closed the "white cloud" fill the lungs completely.

- Suspend breath for a few seconds (three to five) and watch the clean air travel to all extremities of your body.

- Exhale and watch the "smoky de-oxygenated cloud" exit the nostrils as carbon dioxide. See it dissolve and disappear.

- Suspend breath for a few seconds (three to five) and imagine the emptiness of your lungs.

- Repeat this breath-watching process ten or more times and notice the calm relaxation take over.

You are now getting deeper into a Tao Mind state of being, fully relaxed. As this Tao Mind breath-watching process develops, you will become more able to stay unperturbed and totally focused in your centered awareness, in spite of external distractions. Eugene Herrigel wrote in his classic *Zen in the Art of Archery* of how he managed to transcend technique to arrive at this unconscious awareness of the "artless art" of being. Zen is the ideal union of Buddhist meditative mind and Tao Xing, which combines childlike spontaneity and long years of training in the art of self-forgetfulness. In the introduction of Herrigel's book, D. T. Suzuki mentions how this childlikeness is attained "when one thinks yet does not think. One thinks like the showers coming down from the sky; thinks like the waves rolling on the ocean; thinks like the stars illuminating the nightly heavens; he thinks like the green foliage shooting forth in the relaxing spring breeze. Indeed he is the showers, the ocean, the stars, the foliage." No better explanation on Tao Xing can top this description from the Zen master Suzuki!

Once you become comfortable with this technique sitting

down, you can begin to practice it in a standing position and eventually carry this state over to your workout routine and sporting event. It is in this Tao Mind that you will begin to introduce the tools of visual recording (visualization) and affirmation recitation that are detailed in the following two chapters.

After focusing on your breath for ten or so deep inhalations, continue with deep breathing and begin to visualize your workout and/or the athletic activity that you are about to begin. At this point, you may cease watching the breath and focus on the workout. This breath-watching preparation, followed by your visualization and affirmation, will hasten your ability to perform in a calm, efficient, effortless manner, exactly as you would hope to perform.

When you have completed the visualizations and affirmations, take this relaxed state and begin your physical exercise. Start out slowly and maintain your breathing deeply, smoothly, slowly and naturally, for as long as the demands of the physical activity or sport you may be engaging in will allow. You will shift your focus from watching your breath to the task and process at hand. Continue to breathe naturally, deep and full.

Certain sports may demand open mouth breathing occasionally, but in general, breathing through the nostrils is ideal to sustain the full body connection, compared to the "quick panting" alternatives. It takes practice to sustain nostril breathing as your exercise intensifies. However, in time, you will adapt and experience the full benefit of this routine throughout your physical experience. This technique becomes an exhilarating springboard, catapulting you into a more lasting and consistent program for a union between the physical and spiritual in sports, exercise and everyday life.

The Tao Mind approach will help you to see fitness, exercise and sports an internal martial art, a Western yoga, a new Tao and

Zen way of body conditioning. As more of us are working consciously at deeper levels physically, the emotional and spiritual dimensions become inseparable from our whole experience. This Tao Mind simply makes good for playing a good game of life.

Now that you can use breath watching for accessing the Tao Mind in order to create optimal performance prior to all of your physical activity, you can begin to apply this same breathing skill when doing the visualizations and affirmations offered to you in each chapter throughout the five stages on this journey. At the conclusion of each chapter of each stage, we will guide you completely through exercises that will help to reinforce and imprint the message of that chapter into your memory nervous system. In this way, you will ensure its longevity and use on a daily basis in all of your physical and daily activities.

We now lead you to the next chapter in this part, for an overview of the technique of visual recording, or visualization. We will teach you how to develop this skill and use it in various ways as you continue to develop your inner talent.

# Visual Recording

## WHAT YOU SEE, YOU GET

Many hundreds of years ago in ancient China, a celebrated musician was incarcerated by the opposing faction for his participation in a regional uprising. After eight years of solitary confinement, he became a free man. Four weeks into his "new" life, he put on a performance that was judged by his peers to have gone beyond anything he had ever done. Amazed by this, they asked how this could be possible, since he was in an empty cell for so long. He stated that he diligently rehearsed for this concert for hours each day. But he had nothing to practice on, they said. His reply was that although they took his *ch'in*, an ancient zitherlike stringed instrument, they left his mind and all his senses; in his mind's eye, he touched the strings, saw his hands gliding across them, "heard" the intricate melodies, tasted the excitement and felt the heat of his body during and after a deeply sensuous "recital." Amazing? Not really!

The use of visualization techniques for improved performance and cultivating inner mind-sets is not new as evidenced by this story. The disciplines of yoga and meditation from ancient India,

Eastern martial arts and hypnosis are other examples in which the mind's pictures are an integral aspect of one's performance. Today, visualization has found its way into the arenas of sports and exercise where sophisticated athletes, not allowing the outcome of performance to be determined by chance, train the mind and body in synchronous fashion.

Try to imagine yourself on a run; "see," "hear" and "feel" yourself moving. You may even "taste" your salty perspiration and "smell" the air around you. When you visualize in the Tao Mind state, the images become so alive that your central nervous system fails to distinguish between a real or imagined event; your body responds to each in the same way. Thus, when you picture each move of an event correctly in advance , you will have a greater chance of repeating those moves, having in a sense "practiced" them before the actual event. For example, Lee Evans set the world record in the 400-meter race at the 1968 Olympics in Mexico City after two years of daily visualization of each step of the event. Hundreds of other elite and professional athletes create sharp, vivid images of success before they enter the arena. Boxer Muhammad Ali, Olympic diver Greg Louganis, golfer Jack Nicklaus and basketball star Michael Jordan are a few of the greats who have been known to use visualization prior to their stunning performances.

Perhaps one of the most convincing pieces of research to verify the power of imagery in sports was an experiment performed with two groups of basketball players who were trying to improve their free-throw percentage. One group shot one hundred free throws every day for three weeks; the other group simply visualized doing the same. The study found that the visualizing group showed significant improvement over those who actually shot the ball.

Also, when you visualize in the Tao Mind, you will be better able to address your inner demons and concerns more effectively. For example, you can visualize having a setback, feel the disappointment and see yourself responding to the situation in an effective way. Imagine having learned a good lesson from this and feel the exhilaration of going forward in a positive way, once you have benefited from your mistakes. This visualization will help you to grow spiritually and emotionally.

We need to remember that there is a difference between "visual thinking" and the process of visual recording or visualization. The former is a random, unconscious attempt to think about some future event or situation. When left to chance, the thoughts may take the form of negative worry about all of the catastrophic possibilities. Such negative images will create anxiety and fear, increasing the probability of undesirable outcomes.

Visualization, on the other hand, is a planned, conscious use of the "mind's eye" during a deep, relaxed state to create desirable and fulfilling images of a similar future event. It is a form of what you might call "positive worry." You are about to perform in athletics, execute a fitness pattern or take an exam and proceed to "worry" about all of the wonderful possibilities that may occur. Such positive thought patterns will mitigate tension, anxiety and fear, improving the chances for desirable outcomes. This process works by cuing the body to synchronize millions of neural and muscular activities in a dress rehearsal of future events, much like actors getting ready for a stage production. During this process, you call into play as many of your five senses as possible to help you formulate clear, vivid images. By so doing, the pictures developed will be more easily interpreted by the central nervous system "as if" they were real.

The relaxed Tao Mind state helps to stop the "mind chatter" (distractions) and enables you to focus more sharply on the situation being visualized.

Visualization is not magic or hocus-pocus. It is a learned skill that, when practiced regularly in the Tao Mind state, can enable you to focus on what is available to you rather than what you lack. When you "see" limits, they are yours. The idea is to see positive possibilities and dwell on these by selecting images that complement the direction you wish to go or what you wish to do. Of course, visualization will not always provide something that you don't have or are not capable of having. For example, world-class triathlete Mark Allen, winner of numerous Hawaiian Ironman events, like so many elite athletes, relies on visualization techniques to become mentally strong. Recently, with the first race of the season one week away, he realized he was not in the best of physical shape. Rather than panic, he decided to rely on his mental toughness. Each day leading up to the race, he visualized himself as a strong, powerful athlete, racing like the world's best. When he got to the starting line, he felt terrific. Then the race started and "Mike Pigg [his closest rival] went out and kicked my butt. So much for visualization." Allen's story points out that if you don't have what it takes, no amount of brain power will create a miracle. Visualization makes a big difference, however, if you put in the time and physically train. Visualization simply quiets and clears the mind of limiting thoughts and stops it from sabotaging your efforts so that your body is capable of doing what it has been trained to do. For example, you could be the most competent person on the team or candidate for the job. Negative self-talk and images create anxiety and tension, both of which block your efforts to perform up to your capabilities; visualization, on the other hand, clears the way for you to do all that is needed to complete the task successfully. It keeps you on track and maximizes your chances of positive results. It creates expectations of satisfaction, happiness and joy, and you respond by choosing the right people, situations and occurrences that fulfill those expectations. When you carry around images of triumph and success, you create a state of inner calm, confidence and relaxation—all of which contribute to actual success.

If you want to have some fun, try the following exercise:

> To experience the effect of images on muscle response, try lying down with your legs out straight and uncrossed; go to a deep level of relaxation with the Tao Mind. When totally relaxed, imagine your lower legs covered with concrete. "See" the concrete being poured; "feel" the coolness and texture. As it dries, notice how it solidifies and encases your legs. Take another deep breath and, as you exhale, gently try to lift your feet. Don't strain. Be aware of the heaviness of the concrete and how difficult it is to budge that part of your body. Then visualize it crumbling, and feel your legs lifting out from under it, light as air.

Anatomists have shown that images have a powerful impact on every cell of the body. The muscle groups involved in forward motion are activated by images. Visualization enables messages to be sent, on a subliminal level, through your central nervous system to your muscles. Aside from its effect on muscles, visualization—research shows—can actually change blood pressure, heart rate, body temperature and other functions of the body once thought to be solely involuntary physiological processes.

Your mind can be trained like a muscle. If you wanted to build up your body, you wouldn't go to the gym once a month and expect results. So, too, you need to work out mentally with frequency and consistency. Current research suggests that good athletes and other achievers practice their physical *and mental* skills on a daily basis.

Begin to form a habit of using visualization prior to your game or workout to see yourself perform exactly as you would hope. Use it, as well, with the exercises we give to you at the conclusion of each stage chapter. By so doing, you will begin to activate your spiritual talent in the Tao Mind state and put yourself in position for working out and working within. Set aside ten to fifteen minutes a day, to practice. It's best to visualize before eating, or two to three hours after a meal, so that your blood will be in your brain rather than concentrated in your stomach for digestion. When you begin your day with a visualization, the events usually unfold according to your outlook and how you "see" them in your mind's eye.

A question often asked is, "Isn't it dangerous to get my hopes up by visualizing the positive and risk being disappointed? Maybe I should prepare for the worst and if everything turns out okay, great." It's true that preparing for negative possibilities will prevent disappointment, but such thinking also contributes to negative outcomes that weren't necessarily inevitable. Disappointment will not kill; why not increase the likelihood of positive results through the use of visualization?

Here are a few examples of what you may visualize prior to a workout. First imagine your legs very relaxed and loose with the tension flowing away. Imagine your body like a fine-tuned machine. Click into the start of the workout and "see" yourself running, light on your feet. Say to yourself, "This is the best I've ever felt . . . wonderful." Try to imagine various landmarks along the way and see yourself feeling great at each checkpoint. Say to yourself, "I'm so relaxed and so strong I could go another few miles." Notice that the conversation you have with yourself is all positive. Don't say, "I won't get tired"; say, "I remain strong." Also be sure to tell yourself that if your body ever is in danger of doing yourself harm, you'll know to stop rather than cause serious injury. You need this as a precaution against overexertion.

Remember that the conclusion of each chapter will offer you the opportunity to use the sample visualization as a way to nurture, reinforce and solidify the lesson to be learned. Take the opportunity to develop your own personalized visual exercises; go out on a limb, be creative and have fun in the process.

Know that, like any other skill, visualization requires practice. You may master it immediately or need a bit more time to get it down. With patience and practice, you'll be able to create a deep, relaxed Tao Mind state and perform more consistently with positive focus for optimal pleasure, performance and spiritual growth.

You are now ready to go on to the next chapter in this section on cultivating inner talent, the chapter on Affirmation Reciting. As you will discover, affirmations (what you say), are to be used together with visualization (what you see) in order to strengthen your inner talent for working within.

# Affirmation Reciting

## WHAT YOU SAY, YOU DO

A world-class athlete expressed deep concern about her ability to make her third straight U.S. Olympic team. The athletes invited to run the qualifying trials were the best group of runners ever assembled for such a race. Pressure began to build as she verbally told herself, "No way ... I don't deserve to be here. ... There are too many favorites who will make the team before me." It was suggested that she rephrase her negative monologue to one that would reflect the direction she wished to go. She created new phrases: "I am a member of the women's Olympic team"; "I deserve to represent my country at the Olympics"; and "I am in position to strike and get what I like." She was asked to record these sentences on index cards, carry them with her at all times and recite each one a minimum of fifteen times each day and imagine them to be true. After eight months of "marinating" her nervous system with these words, she proceeded to finish first at the trials, making her the fastest and most prominent athlete in her event going into the Olympic games.

According to the Tao, the words you choose are the seeds of

your future realities. The ancient book of Chinese wisdom, the *Tao Te Ching*, says that those who identify with success are welcomed by success; those who identify with failure are likewise welcomed by failure.

In sports, exercise and life, negative thought patterns create mental and physical resistance that greatly hinder performance. Try the following test: hold your arm out straight, while a friend tries to push it down. Resist the pressure as you say out loud, "I love my sport" over and over. Now change the phrase to "I hate my sport" and compare the strength you experience. Notice how much stronger you are, and how much better your performance is, when you vocalize "I love"—a positive thought pattern. How many of us, consciously or not, have a love-hate relationship with sports or exercise. You love the outcome of working out but hate the process. Hate running hills and you'll create greater struggle, making it more difficult to get to the top. Better to say "I love running up hills; they get me into better shape on my way to becoming a better competitor." In this way, you will experience rising up the hill rather than forcing your way there.

Affirmations are very important in the cultivation of inner talent; they are crucial in helping you to awaken to the Tao and living with its influence. Unlike visualization, which controls what you "see," affirmations are the control over what you say. They are strong, positive statements about something that is already true or has the realistic potential for being so. To affirm means "to make firm" by using conscious, planned, positive words and expressions that help to keep you on track with your potential. Without them, the possibility of desirable outcomes diminishes. Affirmations are direct attempts to change patterns of negativity that, like a broken record, continue to repeat themselves. They are words that truly transform the quality of your life, opening you up to the natural way of sports and exercise, the way it was meant to be.

As with visualization, affirmations are practical tools for your success in all situations—in sports, fitness and life—when self-talk becomes damaging. During those times when you are particularly self-critical of your performance or body, consciously choose affirmations that help to alter the negativity. For example, you may repeat often: "I am worthwhile and competent. I deserve the best there is. I have much to offer."

Perhaps you desire to change your physical appearance. Say to yourself, "Slim and trim, I am perfectly fit." By so stating you will create the proper mind-set or environment that will support your willingness to do what's necessary to achieve your image. In this way, affirmations are self-direction, not self-deception; they keep you on track as you continue to approach your goal.

Some of us find it difficult to affirm something that may not be true in the moment. We feel deceitful affirming, "I am a strong and fast athlete," when it may not be so today. However, saying these words will keep your feet pointed in the right direction; you'll be more motivated to do all that's required to reach your goal. Even if you fall short, you will still be further along the path than you would be if you hadn't affirmed your direction in this way. We shouldn't be afraid to open up to the vast possibilities of life.

Affirmations also can be used to help you become more loving, self-accepting, friendly or appreciative, guiding you to greater spiritual expansion; they can help you to develop relationships, become more creative or confident, improve concentration, sharpen your skills or even cope with fatigue. The possibilities are only limited by your imagination.

Affirmations attempt to carry you away from false self-messages and into closer range with your true nature, such as who you are and what is possible given your true self. Affirmations are the language of possibility and change; their purpose is to remove the static, limiting impressions of the mind and create a more unlimited, expansive and abundant sense of self. Affirmations are geared toward the awakening of each of us to our potentialities rather than the limitations of life.

Over the past twenty years I (Jerry) have worked with numerous professional, Olympic and national collegiate champions who, prior to their triumph, have strongly expressed the "I Can't" approach to their upcoming events. My job is to instill in each of them the empowering words "I Can " as a guiding attitude. "I Can" power has directed each one of them on an exciting, fruitful journey of athletic success and satisfaction. When you affirm "I Can," you stimulate the central nervous system with excitement, motivation, courage, confidence, persistence and fearlessness—positive qualities that open the pathways to the unlimited boundaries of your potential.

We suggest that you use the sample affirmations provided with each chapter as well as create personal ones on your own in the space provided underneath those given to you. Also try writing some on three-by-five index cards and strategically mount them in places where they will be visible throughout the day. Place them in a stack and flip through them often; while in a Tao Mind state, visualize what they are saying as you get dressed or get ready for bed. When you create your own, be sure to follow these suggestions to strengthen the words chosen:

- The phrase should be short, pithy, concise, specific and simple.

- It should be positive; affirm what you want, *not* what you don't want. Avoid statements such as "I will *not crash* today." Instead say, "I ride with the skill of a champion."

- Use the present tense. Frame your statements as if the future were now. Rather than "I *will* finish in the top ten," say, "I finish in the top ten." Act "as if" it were true, and it will keep you on track.

- Be consistent. Recite affirmations each day for a few minutes instead of once a week for an hour. A good time to do this is during your visualization session. Picture what the words say.

- Use rhythm. A cadence or rhyme will help you remember a phrase more easily. For example: "I'm in position to *strike* and win on the *bike*."

Remember, within the rose, at all times, is its full potential. It is constantly in the process of change and growth as it comes into its own. When we give it water, sun and nourishment, it blossoms fully. Like this flower, you are a natural unfolding athlete. Nurture yourself with encouragement and positive affirmations avoiding the negative self-talk that kills the spirit. You have all that you need within you now, to become all that you wish. Simply notice that and affirm it to be so.

# PART 2

# Inward Bound

*Entering the*

*Five-Stage*

*Journey for*

*Inner Fitness*

You are now ready for your inward-bound five-stage journey that will change the way you experience sports and exercise. Physical activity will never be the same. At first, you will examine the limits or obstacles that can interfere with your progress and learn ways to hurdle these barriers. Once you do, in Stage 2, you are in position to ignite the passion that you once had as a child and begin to experience a physical resurgence. In Stage 3 of this journey, you will discover ways to expand the boundaries of what you once thought were serious limitations. Overcoming self-imposed limitations will enable you to enter the arena of sports and exercise for the reasons other than battling your opponent, the clock or your physique; in Stage 4, you are now primed to seize your victories from the battle within against the inner demons that block your potential not only in physical activities but in all of life. Finally, in Stage 5, you will begin to use the physical life as a conduit into your deeper self, as a way of meditation and stillness in motion. It is here that you will discover what all poets and philosophers have always known: that the best ideas, thoughts and creations come to you in solitude while in motion. Meet your innermost creative self and begin to find answers to life's most important questions, what life is all about. Each of the following five major stages are subdivided into small, manageable chapters addressing topics that will help you, through stories, anecdotes, meditation, visualization, affirmation and Tao wisdom, to grasp, reinforce, solidify and apply the ancient teachings for becoming internally fit. You will open up to experience not only greater physical performances, but heightened mental, emotional and spiritual dimensions as well. You will begin to feel more alive and childlike. In addition to this, we remind and encourage you to enter the Tao Mind (breath watching, visualizations, affirmations) prior to all physical activity to discover how your workouts can become more effortless in a time devoid of distraction, where life stands still, a period when you can focus on the fun, direction, struggles and joys of your life, and experience enhanced physical performances as well.

*Hurdling the Limits to Discover the Dance*

YUEH

Taking giant strides
Wielding a battle axe
Cutting through all obstructions

*A*t birth, we are all in tune with the Tao, the natural way, a state of complete joy with unlimited potential. Yet almost immediately, society is quick to create boxes for you to fit into, boxes infused with limited beliefs and attitudes that cause you to function far below your capability. Unnecessary fear, unhappiness, timidity, self-doubt, failure, self-deception, struggle and negativity create a conflict with your natural birthright and make it difficult to live up to your potential and obtain what you deserve, a life of well-being, satisfaction and success.

On the first stop of this journey, you begin to hurdle any negative attitudes and barriers you have accumulated over the years that make you resistant to physical activity. For many of us, resistance to such activity happens for many reasons. Perhaps you became derailed by something or someone earlier in life like an insensitive, compassionless, overzealous physical education teacher or coach who insisted upon making you look foolish. Embarrassment early on in the physical-sport realm can throw you off for a lifetime. Being criticized for errors, mistakes or failures can discourage you from ever engaging in sports or fitness. Pressure and anxieties associated with winning and losing, particularly with highly competitive sports, contribute to your demise as an athlete or exercise enthusiast. Fears of success or failure can contribute to waning interest as well.

In this stage, you will learn how to get back to the more natural way, the way of enthusiastic, passionate, childlike play and discover the joy of being fully present in the moment to experience the Zen state of "Satori," the magical dance among body, mind and spirit that makes you feel free to simply let go and have fun. To do this, you will be given the opportunity to look at your fears right from the outset, in the chapter called Facing the Fear. From there, you'll come face to face with the judgmental mind, see what it takes to be open to possibilities, confront the notion of perfection, experience the concept of effortlessness and end with the final chapter in this stage, one that will help you to focus on the dance, the joy, process and fun of sports and exercise.

Many of us forget that all of life is a dance. When you begin to accept this, it becomes possible to choreograph a program of sports and fitness that makes sense, a more natural way as opposed to the normal way of discouragement and failure. Dance with your physical program as you would dance with the deer in the mountains or fish in the lake. A perfect example of nature's dance presented itself to me (Jerry) when I observed my ten-year-old son, Daniel, fishing with his friends. What I noticed was Dan, out on the water in a boat with some terrific kids in a quiet Tao-like environment. I saw passion, love, cooperation, excitement, mentoring, support—the qualities and traits of all healthy relationships engaged in successful endeavors. While there, I observed a sixteen-year-old, his teacher, catch a three-pound bass, kiss it and gently place it back into its home. What I saw was the perfect blend of nature as the boys were "seeking together" (the Latin meaning of the word "competition") the thrill of the catch. No fights, no arguments in this special experience. Here was the dance between human and fish, a peaceful, physical meditation that's rare in our highly competitive world, a world that is limitless and free, where all is possible. The journey that you are now taking, the Tao of Inner Fitness through sports and exercise, gives each of us the opportunity to create a similar dance, one between you and the mountain you run, the bike you ride, the club you swing or the ocean you swim. It is an inward-bound dance, one of aligning and being in concert with nature, free of force, pushing or resisting.

There is nothing you need other than what you already possess to begin to become internally fit. You simply need to be open to a change in the way you see things, a change of attitude and of heart. You need not have special talents or qualities, only an open mind, a Tao mind and the power of "I Can." Assume no limits and begin the dance.

And finally, a few words of reminder: Before each of your daily athletic events or fitness programs, use the breathing and visualization, enter the Tao Mind and envision the activity you are about to begin. Carry the breathing and this state of mind over into your physical regimen for the best results.

# Facing the Fear

According to ancient Taoist wisdom, fear is a catalyst that creates opportunity for movement and growth. When embraced with caution, fear becomes the gateway to spiritual expansion. The Tao encourages against fighting or forcing away fear as this will create inner turmoil, tension and anxiety, all of which interfere with performance of any kind. The Tao teaches us to cooperate with this natural element called fear, blend with it and decipher its message. Like a red light on the dashboard of your car, it warns you of impending danger. It asks the questions: Have you prepared well for what you are doing? Do you have all the information that's required in order to do a good job? Are you performing within your comfort zone? The answers and subsequent corrective actions to these queries usually harness the energy of the fear, enabling you to use it in a constructive way.

When fear shows up as you participate in sports or exercise, see it as a timely opportunity to become more internally fit. Remember that all catastrophic expectations are self-fulfilling prophesies brought on by the fear itself. Whether you fear injury, failure, falling, looking bad or not "making it," rather than moving ahead in this frightened state, allow the fear to instruct you as to what needs to be done. You may be fearful of climbing a steep pitch on the face of a mountain or skiing a double black diamond. Face your inner demon by becoming more skilled through schooling and experience and be thankful for how the fear probably saved your life. Think of ways in which you may get better prepared: more practice, better coaching, safer equipment. By responding to fear in this way you create an important shift in consciousness where you begin to feel a kind of spiritual expansiveness, a freedom that enables you to be more integrated with the Tao, the way things are naturally. With this attitudinal change, you cease to regard fear as a limit, and you focus instead on its sacred value as a guru helping you to progress forward in a safe fashion.

What if your worst fear materialized? You lose the race, fall off your bike or crash on your skis. Even these are moments of inner strengthening and growth. For example, being injured creates unexpected free time, an opportunity for meditation and reflection upon your life and workout program. The mishap provides the chance to reevaluate your situation and possibly make positive beneficial adjustments to what you thought was the perfect setup. When injured, you quickly learn that you can't take your health for granted. You begin to reflect and appreciate your moments of wellness, when you are fit and strong. Injury, for many of us, forces us to grow up and discover an inner strength unknown prior to this setback. The *I Ching*, the Chinese Book of Change and Transformation, tells how reflection brings enlightenment by objectifying your perceptions, helping you to see your situation in an unusual new light. This could be a dynamic time in your life as you explore new ideas, experiences, careers and opportunities.

The same Tao wisdom applies to fear in all of life. When confronted with fear of any kind, embrace it cautiously and wait until you feel more comfortable before forging ahead. It helps to communicate your fears with others who have had similar feelings and successfully handled them. This can put it into perspective and help to mitigate the fear.

You will also notice how often your fear is the result of standing at the doorway of an enormous task: searching for a new job, finishing an advanced educational degree, writing a book. Being overwhelmed by such undertakings creates fright; it helps to follow the Tao and its teachings about moderation: Do less yet achieve more. Divide a task into small manageable segments in order to reduce this fear. For example, at mile eighteen of a marathon with eight to go, you may panic and become quite anxious. Focus not on running eight miles, but on only one and run it eight times. That's less frightening and more relaxing, thus making it easier to complete the task, free of the debilitating fear.

As you learn to apply these Taoist principles, your "fear comfort zone" will grow wider and your physical world will continue to provide opportunity to strengthen your inner fitness. For example, what was frightening to you last year may now seem less intimidating; you're more comfortable with a task that once created enormous fear. You are more emotionally and spiritually aligned with a concept that, at one time, created great havoc. Fear is, indeed, your sacred friend.

Use the following exercises to help you cultivate inner talent and to nurture and reinforce facing your fear. Remember, also, that you will want to precede your daily workout or sports activity with a ten-minute Tao Mind breathing and visualization session to help you relax and focus on how you wish to perform your exercise regimen:

## A.  BREATH WATCHING

- Inhale slowly through the nostrils and watch with your eyes closed the "white cloud" fill the lungs completely.

- Suspend breath for a few seconds (three to five) and watch the clean air travel to all extremities of your body.

- Exhale and watch the "smoky de-oxygenated cloud" exit the nostrils as carbon dioxide. See it dissolve and disappear.

- Suspend breath for a few seconds (three to five) and imagine the emptiness of your lungs.

- Repeat this breath-watching process ten or more times and notice the calm relaxation take over.

## B.  VISUALIZATION

Now in your relaxed Tao Mind state, keep your eyes closed and:

- *Invite* your fear to "sit" with you and talk.

- *Say,* "Hi there, Fear. I appreciate your teaching me to become a better athlete [speaker, teacher, parent, coach]. What do I need to know or do to improve?"

- *Listen* to the response and see yourself following the advice of the companion.

- *See* this "tiger" become an amiable cat.

- *Embrace* the "tiger" and begin to gain inner strength.

- *Feel* the fear dissipate when you begin to do what's necessary to become confident.

- *See* yourself moving ahead with joy and certainty that all is good.

## C. AFFIRMATIONS

Remember that the following are samples of affirmations that reinforce the Tao lesson to be learned. On the blank lines provided, create some affirmations that are more personal and relevant to your journey. Experiment and have fun in the process and make good use of index cards, posting your affirmations in a variety of places. Also recite them to yourself during visualization, and picture what the words actually say.

Hello, Fear. I am listening.

Fear is natural, a welcome challenge.

I am okay knowing fear is with me.

Fear, let's be friends.

_____

_____

_____

## D. APPLICATION OF ANCIENT WISDOM

Use the following pragmatic shifts in attitude to help restructure your conceptual view of the world around you:

> *Be sure to face your fear directly, square in the eye. Instead of superficially hoarding security blankets for protection, learn to relinquish these old tricks of temporary psychological relief. By shifting your attitude, you can turn the paralysis of numbing dullness into adrenal stimulus to improve your performance. Acknowledge the positive phenomenon of having "butterflies in the stomach"; this feeling can ensure an inspired and surprisingly fresh performance. The potent metaphor, Embrace the Tiger, in Tai Ji practice is exactly created for this learning. This beast embodies the multidimensional power of blinding beauty, ruthless strength, godlike passion as well as the gentle and loving quality of the lamb. This shifted Tao concept transforms the fierce and frightful into innocence and light. Embrace your Tiger!*

# Thinking Mind, Judging Mind

In the Chinese Book of Change and Transformation, the *I Ching*, you are encouraged to cultivate only productive attitudes toward yourself, since you are the product of everything you put into your mind. All performance in sports, exercise and life is a strong reflection of your self-talk. Like the Tao, you are a natural process, and if you ignore this ancient natural law, you set yourself up for misery and failure.

When we encounter self-critical athletes, we ask them if they would talk to their friends in the same way. "Absolutely not!" they usually reply. We encourage them to be as friendly to themselves as they are to their friends in such situations. Self-criticism has the same effects as criticism of others; it makes you begin to distrust yourself; you lose confidence in your ability to perform.

This happened to an All-American candidate in tennis, following a devastating defeat. According to him, he was sloppy, slow, not good enough and probably should avoid the national championships. His performance for the next month reflected his self-talk and he was on the verge of giving up his sport. His coach pointed out to him how his disappointing tennis was an opportunity to see his situation as an internal crisis from which he could not only improve his game but also grow as a person. Tennis became his path to self-discovery, and he began to use his game to better understand himself and to learn how he stood in his own way of achieving greatness. This shift in consciousness enabled him to stop the self-abuse and find compassion through the use of positive affirmations. His newly found inner-fitness approach enabled him to relax and perform at higher levels in the hostility-free internal environment he had created. His self-compassion had a ripple effect on his team as well. According to the ancient Chinese notion of the "ripple effect," when you drop a pebble in the water, everything that comes within the water's wake is directly affected by it. From his own inner peaceful environment, he enabled those around him to perform in a more relaxed way.

Negative mind-sets block your progress by inhibiting your courage, confidence, concentration and enthusiasm for sports and fitness. Ultimately, the hypercritical mind will discourage you entirely from participating in any physically related activity. As of now, only fifteen percent of the adult population participates in any kind of sport, fitness or exercise-related program. This astoundingly small percentage is due in large part to criticism induced from insensitive coaches, teachers, parents and themselves. We have known for centuries that you are the product of your environment, what it says about you and what your mind thinks about the comments.

To get a sense of how a judging mind impacts you physically, emotionally and spiritually, recite these words over and over, out loud: "I am a worthless, out-of-shape, unathletic loser." Now notice how you feel when you say, "I am an extremely fit, strong, vibrant, talented athlete." Now extend your arm firmly and ask someone to push it down as you recite each phrase individually. Try to resist each time your arm is pushed. Notice how much stronger you are when you choose words that validate, not criticize. Notice, also, how you feel in your heart and spirit when you engage in a more positive, nonjudgmental mind.

Sports and exercise are perfect environments that provide an opportunity to observe what happens when you create a "dancing mind," a nonjudgmental Tao mind. When you catch yourself being the critical judge during a workout or game, let go of the negative comments and become aligned with the Tao, a more natural way, by saying, "Here I am, doing my favorite thing in the world, just trying to have some fun." Follow this statement with a quick image of performing well with extreme joy and satisfaction. Notice how quickly your mood shifts and your spirit comes alive.

In order to help yourself, write a list of your own put-downs (I'm not good enough, I don't deserve, I'm too old . . . too fat . . . slow) that you recite with regard to your sport or physical life. Then immediately create a list of opposite, positive statements that contradict the negative. You now have a list of affirmations that, when recited on a regular daily basis, will direct you toward your best emotional, spiritual and physical self.

Use the following exercises to help you cultivate and strengthen your inner talent and to nurture and reinforce positive self-talk. Remember, also, that you will want to precede your daily workout or sports activity with a ten-minute Tao Mind breathing and visualization session to help you relax and focus on how you wish to perform your exercise regimen:

## A. BREATH WATCHING

- Inhale slowly through nostrils and watch with your eyes closed the "white cloud" fill the lungs completely.

- Suspend breath for a few seconds (three to five) and watch the clean air travel to all extremities of your body.

- Exhale and watch the "smoky de-oxygenated cloud" exit the nostrils as carbon dioxide. See it dissolve and disappear.

- Suspend breath for a few seconds (three to five) and imagine the emptiness of your lungs.

- Repeat this breath-watching process ten or more times and notice the calm relaxation take over.

## B. VISUALIZATION

Again, in your relaxed Tao Mind state, keep eyes closed and:

- *See* yourself "write" words that portray you negatively on paper.

- *Look* at the words on the sheet; then crumple it up into a ball.

- *Strike* a match, in your mind's eye, and set the ball on fire.

- *Watch* it disintegrate into ashes and be blown away by the wind, forever.

- *See* yourself "write" words that nurture your spirit.

- *Place* them in visible places throughout your home and "hear" yourself recite them.

- *Feel* the strength you gain when changing to the more positive words.

- *See* yourself as a vibrant, dancing athlete and human being, full of life.

## C. AFFIRMATIONS

Remember that the following are samples of affirmations that reinforce the Tao lesson to be learned. On the blank lines provided, create some affirmations that are more personal and relevant to your journey. Experiment and have fun in the process and make good use of index cards, posting your affirmations in a variety of places. Also recite them to yourself during visualization and picture what the words actually say.

I say YES! to all my potentials.

I challenge myself to be the best I can be.

I have within me all that I need to have my wish come true.

I am a joyful, smiling, dancing spirit.

_____

_____

_____

## D. APPLICATION OF WISDOM

Use the following pragmatic shifts in attitude to help restructure your conceptual view of the world around you:

*Remember, nature is spontaneous, noninterfering, ever-changing and accepting. It is without judgment. Learn to trust your personal power, your integrity. When you feel self-critical, return to the heart-mind unity and proceed in your daily sport or workout without undue stress and conflict. Your Tao nature refuses to be critical or judgmental. Your body-mind thinks and dances as a whole, unimpeded. We suggest that you contemplate the eight Tao philosophical tenets in the section on the philosophy of Tao in Part I to receive added support and direction to change this concept of the judging mind to a more open, receptive Tao Mind.*

# The Power of "I Can"

We are reminded by the *Tao Te Ching* how advanced individuals have no fixed minds. The Tao teaches you to be flexible with beliefs, as rigidity will block your growth. Fixed mind-sets such as "I can't . . ." obscure the unlimited boundaries of your potential. This ancient wisdom also recommends the importance of renouncing your restrictive beliefs about what you can and cannot do in life. Know that your strength as an athlete or fitness enthusiast begins when you shift your consciousness to the notion of abundance and fortify yourself with "I Can" power.

At this point on the journey, open up to the Tao mind where you accept a host of new attitudes and possibilities that encourage you to move forward, free of the "I can't" philosophy. To not do this is to have a fixed, rigid mind that makes for rigid bodies and tight, inflexible performances in sports, exercise and all arenas of life.

The words "I can't . . ." are usually based on subjective evidence, nothing more. Unless you have tried, you probably cannot formulate a belief as to what you can or can't do. Believing "you can't" will keep you blind to any possibilities of discovering how you can. This is best exemplified by the allegory of "the magic wishing box":

> A middle-aged man hoped to meet someone with whom to share his life. Although he wanted this, he didn't really believe "I Can." He mentioned this to a good friend, who suggested that he visit a certain palm reader who had tremendous success helping people create meaningful relationships. The man agreed to do it. When he and the palm reader met, she gave him a magic black box and instructed him to write his wish on a piece of tissue paper and deposit it into the box, and a new person would come into his life. He believed her, followed the directions and, shortly thereafter, met the most incredible woman, fell in love and married her six months later. He went back to the palm reader to share his joy and thank her for the magic box, asking her how it worked. She quickly explained: "There's no such thing as a magic box. The magic was in your believing that you can."

We are reminded of those well-chosen words of inventor Henry Ford: "Whether you believe you can or believe you can't—you're probably right." When you believe "I Can," you create the opportunity for attitudinal shifts. These two simple words enable you to discover within the day's passion, hope, determination, faith, motivation, commitment, confidence, concentration and excitement, all feelings of the soul that turn you on to greater, more satisfying possibilities, not only in sports, but life as well. Thinking "I can't" dampens and kills the spirit and sabotages any efforts or attempts to acquire what you deserve.

What we notice about our work, with elite Olympic, professional and collegiate athletes, is that those who do the best seem to possess certain mind-sets in common. They "think" like champions, and assume that "I Can."

> She was a twenty-year-old mother of a two-year-old, and one of twenty-two children born to a struggling family in rural America. As a child, she was afflicted with polio, told by her doctors that she'd probably never walk normally without a brace. In and out of hospitals for much of her early years, this ordinary person never lost her spirit; she believed that "I Can" overcome this crippling disease. In miraculous fashion, she became the first female to win three gold medals in an Olympics. Her name is Wilma Rudolph.

Like Wilma, you are an ordinary person capable of extraordinary things; you simply need to believe "I Can" and apply yourself accordingly. Say "I Can," then take a sacred journey, searching for the truth; collect the data that substantiates this power statement. This new Tao mind-set will enable you to feel alive and unlock the extraordinary potential that you inherently possess.

In athletics and fitness regimes, as with most of life, many of us decide, before we even try, what we can or can't do. Try not to be so rigid; when you feel yourself getting tight, try to keep a soft, flexible mind and believe that all is possible until the data comes back to prove otherwise.

A national-class runner was hurting badly at mile twenty-three of a marathon. Rather than give up, he told himself "I can do this" and dug down deep to see what he had left. By claiming "I can," he found hidden reserves and discovered how to work with his fear, fatigue and self-doubt. These sacred teachings have enabled him to continue a forward direction when, professionally, he tires after five intensive days of teaching or when he faces the final phases of editorial changes with his books or when life seems out of control as the father of three young testosterone-filled boys.

Now, choose an activity that appeals to you and begin to challenge your spirit by doing things you'd like, but to which you historically have said "I can't do that." Perhaps it's a class in dance, drumming, martial arts or yoga. Maybe you have always wanted to sky dive or water-ski. Perhaps you'd like to enter a race and compete in your age category. All of those require you to take action and approach your fears; remember the first chapter? By saying "I Can," you'll feel empowered and so alive especially when you discover that you truly "can do it." Self-image, a concept of deep inner concern for most of us, will be greatly enhanced in the process. Remember that most of us can change the way we feel about ourselves by simply changing the beliefs of our minds. On this journey, put your mind into the "I Can" state, your ultimate power to alter not only your physical life, but the bigger game of life as well.

Use the following exercises to help you cultivate inner talent and to nurture and reinforce the power of "I Can." Remember, also, that you will want to precede your daily workout or sports activity with a ten-minute Tao Mind breathing and visualization session to help you relax and focus on how you wish to perform your exercise regimen:

## A.  BREATH WATCHING

Again, in our relaxed Tao Mind state, with eyes closed:

- Inhale slowly through nostrils and watch with your eyes closed the "white cloud" fill the lungs completely.

- Suspend breath for a few seconds (three to five) and watch the clean air travel to all extremities of your body.

- Exhale and watch the "smoky de-oxygenated cloud" exit the nostrils as carbon dioxide. See it dissolve and disappear.

- Suspend breath for a few seconds (three to five) and imagine the emptiness of your lungs.

- Repeat this breath-watching process ten or more times and notice the calm relaxation take over.

## B.  VISUALIZATION

Again, in your relaxed Tao Mind state, with eyes closed:

- *Choose* a situation or task in which you've told yourself: "I can't do that; it's too hard."

- *See* yourself taking it on and performing exactly as you would like.

- *Feel* exhilarated as your performance goes beyond belief; your confidence soars.

- *Feel* proud of taking the huge steps and believing in yourself, regardless of the outcome.

- *Be* open to the vast possibilities available to you.

## C. AFFIRMATIONS

Remember that the following are samples of affirmations that reinforce the Tao lesson to be learned. On the blank lines provided, create some affirmations that are more personal and relevant to your journey. Experiment and have fun in the process and make good use of index cards, posting your affirmations in a variety of places. Also recite them to yourself during visualization and picture what the words actually say.

What I believe, I usually receive.

I can become whatever I visualize.

I possess "I Can" Power.

Why Not?

_____

_____

_____

## D.    APPLICATION OF ANCIENT WISDOM

Use the following pragmatic shifts in attitude to help restructure your conceptual view of the world around you:

> Use the earth below as a grounding device to regain the powerful sense of security and well-being. Then concentrate deep inside on the fire burning in your belly. This is the "Can" place to plug into. Close your eyes as you sit or stand securely and firmly, and place both hands right on your belly. Breathe deeply and feel the power. See the fire of life burning bright, and say, "HA!" Repeat, "I Can. Yes, I Can." And, "HA! HA! HA!" Now go on with your workout.

# Yield to the Unachievable

To strive for perfection is, in itself, an act of imperfection. It is an attempt to achieve the unachievable. Tao wisdom encourages you to yield to your tendency to be perfect; when you do, the anxiety, stress and tension caused by your futile attempts at the impossible will be reduced, you will feel better, and your performance will improve. Also, you will recapture the joy, fulfillment and passion of sports and exercise as you enter this magical arena with the pure spirit of play, without having to be what you can't be—perfect. Yielding to the unachievable in sports and exercise trains you to develop a deeper inner sense of compassion as you begin to understand that you live in a world where even the greatest of athletes are imperfect. Babe Ruth struck out more than 1,300 times in a sport where batting .300 is considered great, yet a far cry from perfect. Paradoxically, when you become spiritually fortified with compassion for your shortcomings, you begin to get closer to perfection.

John Wooden, former coach of the UCLA Bruin basketball dynasty, knows something about this. His teams dominated the NCAA basketball scene for fifteen years, winning numerous national championships. Yet he never harped on maintaining perfect records, even during an undefeated season. He realized that each season was imperfect and had its share of problems and challenges. He knew that the stress and tension from trying to be undefeated would have caused great anxiety in his athletes.

Then there's the wonderful success story of Georgetown University head coach John Thompson during the NCAA basketball championship game against North Carolina. Georgetown, playing a near perfect game, had a chance for victory in the finals when Fred Brown of GU mistook an opposing player for a teammate and threw him the ball. That iced the game for Carolina and big (six-foot-ten) John, his coach, walked over to his athlete, put his long arms around Brown, held and consoled him. He told Brown that no one is perfect and that without him, they wouldn't even have reached the finals. John's heartfelt compassion following a tremendous loss created enormous unity and loyalty among his players. Two years later, GU won the NCAA championship with Thompson as a coach who asks for excellence, not perfection. Psychologically and emotionally the team was unlimited because of his actions. According to the *Tao Te Ching*, efforts to be perfect are actually psychological and spiritual limits that we place upon ourselves.

As you begin to take the Tao of Inner Fitness journey, it would be most helpful to shift your consciousness and yield to the temptation to achieve perfection. The journey will be much less painful if you do. A Tao Mind approach helps you to see how all athletes, all humans make mistakes and are, by definition, imperfect beings. So, therefore, it's perfect to be imperfect. To be perfect is inconsistent with being human; perfection belongs to the gods.

Perfection is simply a guide to keep you on track, heading in the direction of self-improvement. It is not meant to be a goal or a place to reach. When you find yourself in sports or exercise trying to be perfect or getting down on yourself for not being so, tell yourself that this is futile folly, an attempt to achieve the unachievable. Be kind to yourself and try to do the best you can with what you've got. Then imagine yourself performing with excellence, and feel good about your choice. The idea is to shoot for perfection, knowing, at all times, that you will fall short; yet, because of the effort, you'll be further along than you might have been had you not had such a lofty goal from the start. When you do this, you need to remember to exhibit self-compassion and not measure your self-worth as an athlete or a person by the outcome. You can be great at anything, and be imperfect at the same time.

When you make a mistake, see it as your physical life giving you the opportunity to further your inner fitness; you're learning to have a kind heart and develop the flexibility to see imperfection for what it truly is. When you shoot for perfection in sports, fitness and life, become soft in your attitudes and yield to it; don't fight it and you'll go forward. Remember that, according to the Tao, soft is, indeed, strong. By releasing the need to be perfect, you reduce anxiety and tension and begin to feel good about yourself in all aspects of sports and life.

As a suggestion, replace perfection (an outcome-oriented concept) with excellence (a process-based concept), which refocuses your attention inward on higher pursuits such as pride, self-esteem, courage, perseverance, satisfaction and fun in the execution of a well-thought-out plan, or a particular mechanical skill. Your self-worth should always be gauged by the process of how you "play the game," on and off the court. Results therefore, become the by-products of this successful inner soul-based process.

Use the following exercises to help you cultivate inner talent and to nurture and reinforce the process of excellence. Remember, also, that you will want to precede your daily workout or sports activity with a ten-minute Tao Mind breathing and visualization session to help you relax and focus on how you wish to perform your exercise regimen:

## A. BREATH WATCHING

Again, in our relaxed Tao Mind state, with eyes closed:

- Inhale slowly through nostrils and watch with your eyes closed the "white cloud" fill the lungs completely.

- Suspend breath for a few seconds (three to five) and watch the clean air travel to all extremities of your body.

- Exhale and watch the "smoky de-oxygenated cloud" exit the nostrils as carbon dioxide. See it dissolve and disappear.

- Suspend breath for a few seconds (three to five) and imagine the emptiness of your lungs.

- Repeat this breath-watching process ten or more times and notice the calm relaxation take over.

## B. VISUALIZATION

Again, in your relaxed Tao Mind state, with eyes closed:

- *Choose* a project at work or at home.

- *See* yourself doing excellent work.

- *Feel* the annoyance and letdown from making a mistake.

- *Judge* yourself as incompetent, then—

- *Say:* "Stop."

- *Validate* yourself by saying, "I am a very capable, competent person."

- *Learn* from the setback and forge ahead to completion.

- *Feel* relaxed, calm and satisfied as you do excellent work to completion.

## C. AFFIRMATIONS

Remember that the following are samples of affirmations that reinforce the Tao lesson to be learned. On the blank lines provided, create some affirmations that are more personal and relevant to your journey. Experiment and have fun in the process and m good use of index cards, posting your affirmations in a variety of places. Also recite them to yourself during visualization and picture what the words actually say.

I see the natural beauty of what it is, the way it is.

I have the perfect vision to guide my imperfection along.

My imperfection is a springboard for my continual growth.

_____

_____

_____

## D.  APPLICATION OF ANCIENT WISDOM

Use the following pragmatic shifts in attitude to help restructure your conceptual view of the world around you:

*No use struggling upstream; push the river and waste your energy. When you feel defeated from a less than perfect performance, switch your perspective to a more positive note. If the wind blows you over, become the wind. When the waves are too strong, become the ocean. Catch the wind and sail, instead of rowing the boat breathlessly. Dive into the center of the waves to be carried along. Spread your wings to ride the wind. These are all typical Tai Ji moves that set your mind dancing and propel your body into action. Everything seems possible. Embody these principles in your whole being and blend with nature's imperfections.*

# Effort Without Effort

Vince Stroth, a student of Tao and an offensive guard for the Houston Oilers, was asked how he could continually survive the vicious pounding he got from the opposition. He said that he made the effort to work according to his game plan: He effortlessly takes the oncoming defensive player and diverts his force to the side rather than opposing it. The harder his opponent's attack, the less effort it is for him to direct his force to the ground, away from the ball.

The ancient Chinese book of Change and Transformation, the *I Ching*, talks about the wisdom of using four ounces to deflect four thousand pounds. Seems as though Vince knew this. The Tao continues to remind us how the most flexible parts of the world overcome the most rigid. In *The Art of War*, his classic book on conflict strategy, Sun Tzu strongly recommends that we follow the way of least effort. In Chinese, this effortless effort state is called Wu Wei, meaning "do not do that which is not natural." It's not natural to push, force or fight the flow. It is more productive and peaceful to go with the flow and move in accordance with what nature provides. Make the effort to exert less effort.

You see it constantly in sports and exercise. When you decide to cut back, let up and exert less effort, your performance begins to improve. This principle of effortless effort was successfully demonstrated by Olympic runners Ray Norton, Tommie Smith, John Carlos and Lee Evans. Their coach, Bud Winter, developed the ninety percent law. When runners try to perform at one hundred percent, they get anxious and tense. Too much effort blocks their Qi flow, their life energy force, and diminishes their power. Performing at nine-tenths effort is more relaxing and results in faster speed.

Let's say you're trying to run up a steep hill. The more effort you exert, the more difficult it seems to be. Rather than apply effort, enjoy the natural surroundings and try to glide rather than push yourself up. Rigidity sets in when anything reaches its full limit. When you do your weight training, for example, relax your muscles yet keep your arms firm as you lift. Notice how much stronger you feel by not exerting as much. All of your physical activity will go up a notch as you begin to exert less. This is easily demonstrated by doing push-ups. Get in position, relax your arms and face, and effortlessly do two of them. Now, repeat the process using tensed arms. Notice how much easier it is when you apply less force, effort and push. Maybe we should call them "rise-ups."

When you learn the advantage of paying attention to the energy flow and rhythms in your sports and exercise program and see how pushing or forcing is counterproductive, you begin to apply this notion of the effortless effort to the rest of life. Often times your inner turmoil, struggle and pain are the result of your continual effort to force what cannot be. You quickly enter a spiritual vacuum as frustration, anger, depression and fear begin to take over as a result of your futile attempts to control the uncontrollable. A strong feeling of inner peace is the inevitable result of practicing Wu Wei, action with the sense of going with the flow.

When you find yourself forcing and exerting to finish a project, you increase the chance of getting stuck. Authors are famous for getting "writer's block" when they try too hard to be creative. When blockage happens, focus on the inner spiritual elements of joy, beauty and the flow of your art. Give attention to the results and notice how much better you feel about your work as it begins to go more smoothly. Tell yourself that you're simply here to enjoy the task, and don't perseverate on the outcome. Ask yourself, "How can I do it more effortlessly?" Then follow your advice. You practically have to "not care" yet not be totally "care-less" in this delicate balance of effortless effort.

Notice the peace you experience when you choose to step aside as tension mounts, rather than to force your opinion on others; when you choose to enter a relationship and not force the process; when you choose not to push for an unnaturally speedy recovery when sick or injured. Martial artists have understood for centuries that the less effort you exert, the more proficient and spiritually sane you will become in all that you do.

Use the following exercises to help you cultivate deep inner talent and to nurture and reinforce effortless effort. Remember, also, that you will want to precede your daily workout or sports activity with a ten-minute Tao Mind breathing and visualization session to help you relax and focus on how you wish to perform your exercise regimen:

## A.  BREATH WATCHING

Again, in our relaxed Tao Mind state, with eyes closed:

- Inhale slowly through nostrils and watch with your eyes closed the "white cloud" fill the lungs completely.

- Suspend breath for a few seconds (three to five) and watch the clean air travel to all extremities of your body.

- Exhale and watch the "smoky de-oxygenated cloud" exit the nostrils as carbon dioxide. See it dissolve and disappear.

- Suspend breath for a few seconds (three to five) and imagine the emptiness of your lungs.

- Repeat this breath-watching process ten or more times and notice the calm relaxation take over.


## B.  VISUALIZATION

Again, in your relaxed Tao Mind state, with eyes closed:

- *Take* on a task—sports, exercise or professionally related— that usually requires a huge effort.

- *See* yourself going about it with effortlessness.

- *Feel* a lightness about it and refuse to obsess about the level of difficulty.

- *Experience* yourself exerting less effort as you glide or float through the task.

- *Feel* relaxed yet efficient, smooth, strong.

- *Notice* how it seems so easy, yet your level of performance has improved.

- *Feel* a keen sense of finishing a job and doing it well.

## C. AFFIRMATIONS

Remember that the following are samples of affirmations that reinforce the Tao lesson to be learned. On the blank lines provided, create some affirmations that are more personal and relevant to your journey. Experiment and have fun in the process and make good use of index cards, posting your affirmations in a variety of places. Also recite them to yourself during visualization and picture what the words actually say.

I gain more as I exert less.

With a relaxed body-mind, I care less and can do more.

Breathing in, breathing out, I am doing just fine.

Wu Wei all the way!

_____

_____

_____

## D. APPLICATION OF ANCIENT WISDOM

Use the following pragmatic shifts in attitude to help restructure your conceptual view of the world around you:

*Review the philosophy of Wu Wei in Part I. Imagine becoming one with the horse, riding bareback, feeling the galloping grace of this wild animal without reducing and controlling its powerful potential by strapping and harnessing.*

*Here again, distinguish between sailing and rowing, downhill skiing and mountain climbing, surfing and water-skiing, dragged behind a motorboat.*

# Enjoying the Dance

Once again, the *I Ching* provides us with the encouragement to attend to the dance, the process rather than the product. When you center your attention in the moment and act in harmony with the times, you will experience much inner peace and fulfillment. According to the Tao, by staying in the present, you can do less yet gain more; you create more personal power and energy, enabling you, paradoxically, to have greater influence over the outcome.

When most of us begin a sport or exercise program, our motivations and reasons for participating are usually narrow and specific. The universal, more infinite aspects are rarely understood. When you enjoy the dance, you help to widen and expand your focus and create a bridge between the physical and spiritual so that sports and exercise can touch every aspect of your being. Think about the following metaphor:

> Euro- and Native Americans, upon coming across a herd
> of deer in the wilderness, display quite different reactions.
> The first thing Euro-Americans do is count the number of

deer in the herd, as if this outcome contributed something significant to the situation. The Native Americans, on the other hand, would gaze at the herd for hours observing, perhaps, their place of origin and comment on their destination. If you asked for a numerical report on that same herd, they would appear dumbfounded. To the Native American, the spiritual intangibles of joy, satisfaction and fulfillment are the result of being in the process of what is happening; the beauty is the dance itself.

Many of us are so preoccupied with the outcomes, results, mechanical and technical aspects of our game and life that we overlook the fun or the reason why we play, rushing instead, to reach a goal, as if that were the purpose of playing or participating.

We sense that much of the resistance you may feel toward physical activity and sports has to do with the pressures and tensions related to pushing for outcomes and results. When you feel this way, know that the key to maintaining your passion for this particular physical life is to come back to the essence of the game or experience itself, be in the moment and enjoy the beauty of the activity.

This point is clearly exhibited by two friends playing tennis. Jack, a one-time nationally ranked athlete, is quite serious about his game, plays daily and takes pride in his reputation for victories against tough opponents. Jim takes a more Zen approach to his game, one of floating the ball over the net as he choreographs the dance between him and his opponent. Contented to keep the play at that level, Jim gets annoyed by his "serious tennis" partner who pushes to play a set and keep score. Jim "gives in" to the request. Forcing his shots in hopes of winning every point, Jack becomes frustrated and angry as Jim safely returns each ball in his "Tai Ji tennis" way, floating and dancing around the court. Jim, feeling peaceful, calm, and joyous, easily wins in two sets 6–1, 6–0, completely baffling Jack.

When you find yourself being ruled by the scores and outcomes of your physical tasks, build a stronger, more sublime base; focus on the process and appreciate each moment of play. You can do this by asking the question: "Why am I doing this . . . really?" Get in touch with your inner, deeper motives for entering this particular arena of sports and fitness—why you play the game. You'll discover that much of it has little to do with the outcome or the product. It is the process, joy, satisfaction and fun in the execution of a particular skill or move that turns you on. There is a strong divine connection between you and your sport. This is the dance that we refer in which you totally give in to the natural movement of your physical routine. No need to think; silence the conscious mind. Put all aside; just play and dance the dance.

This narrow focus, one of complete absorption in the task, is felt by many elite athletes and can be experienced by you. Danny Ferry, a star basketball athlete for the NBA Cleveland Cavaliers, describes his experience with the dance as "a quiet, peaceful state where I am completely unaware of the shouting spectators; it's a magical zone where all goes right, a complete absorption in what I'm doing, a flowing state without any need to control and a trance-like feeling where all things move along smoothly and naturally, as if they were perfect." His description followed a career-best thirty-four-point performance against the New York Knicks.

Developing the power to be in the moment is a valuable skill in sports as well as other events in life. One way to accomplish this task is to block out the external distractions by narrowing your focus to some minute detail. Your central nervous system enjoys working with smaller targets.

For example, if you are a competitive rower, hear the splash of the oar as it paddles the water. If you are a baseball athlete, try to keep your eye on the ball by focusing on the seam as the ball leaves the pitcher's hand; if you are a runner, tune in to your form, pace and fluid movement; concentrate on your golf club, lacrosse stick or bicycle as if they were natural extensions of your body. If you are a golfer, "park" your attention on the ball's brand name and try to see the club face strike it cleanly. As a tennis athlete, see each point as a new beginning and repeat over and over the word "hit" precisely when the ball does hit the ground. When shooting a foul shot in basketball, focus on the front of the rim and see the perfect rotation of the seams on the ball as it cleanly slips over it for a score. When doing breath-watching exercises, focus on the inhalation as a white cloud entering the nasal passageways, into the lungs and penetrating the entire body.

The same principle applies to daily life. Whether you are cooking, cleaning house, or planting flowers, try to concentrate on the textures, the smells, colors, tastes, sounds, all Zen moments of focused joy. When distracted, take a few deep breaths and return to one small aspect of the task. All of this requires practice and time. The next time you are cleaning up after dinner, get into the dance of washing the plates—the Tao of dishes as it were.

Take these lessons from your sport and physical activity and apply them to what you do in life. Become more conscious about your inner, deeper reasons for following your path. By so doing, you will open your life to the possibility of more enjoyment, passion and love. For example, there was a miserable, unhappy man who had a healthy income selling a not so healthy product—tobacco. When he focused on the money, he was temporarily satisfied. Knowing that he was selling something that contributed to global illness, however, created enough cognitive dissonance that he suffered emotionally each day. He wasn't enjoying his dance. Eventually, he changed his emphasis about work: He decided to empty his pockets to fill his soul. Although he didn't earn as much financially, he became immeasurably wealthy, feeling good about himself and the heartfelt work he chose as a counselor with emotionally challenged youths.

The key to keeping the fires of passion flaming well into the night—in sports, exercise or any arena of life—is to be sure you enjoy the dance. When you focus on the beauty and essence of the game, activity or what you do, you will cease to experience the anxiety and pressures related to outcomes and results and contribute to your overall level of inner fitness. You will feel good all over.

Use the following exercises to help you cultivate inner talent and to nurture and reinforce the process and dance. Remember, also, that you will want to precede your daily workout or sports activity with a ten-minute Tao Mind breathing and visualization session to help you relax and focus on how you wish to perform your exercise regimen:

## A.  BREATH WATCHING

Again, in our relaxed Tao Mind state, with eyes closed:

- Inhale slowly through nostrils and watch with your eyes closed the "white cloud" fill the lungs completely.

- Suspend breath for a few seconds (three to five) and watch the clean air travel to all extremities of your body.

- Exhale and watch the "smoky de-oxygenated cloud" exit the nostrils as carbon dioxide. See it dissolve and disappear.

- Suspend breath for a few seconds (three to five) and imagine the emptiness of your lungs.

- Repeat this breath-watching process ten or more times and notice the calm relaxation take over.


## B. VISUALIZATION

Again, in your relaxed Tao Mind state, with eyes closed:

- *Visualize* yourself engaged in a game or physical activity.

- *Notice* all the distraction.

- *Focus* on one small aspect of the activity—the writing on the ball, for example.

- *Say* the word "flow" over and over.

- *Feel* yourself free of tension, relaxed and floating.

- *See* your performance as an easy, flowing experience.

- *Feel* in sync. It's only you and the game.

## C.  AFFIRMATIONS

Remember that the following are samples of affirmations that rein-force the Tao lesson to be learned. On the blank lines provided, create some affirmations that are more personal and relevant to your journey. Experiment and have fun in the process and make good use of index cards, posting your affirmations in a variety of places. Also recite them to yourself during visualization and pic-ture what the words actually say.

> Focus on the steps, on the flow, dance on.
>
> Now is the moment, enjoy.
>
> I am the dancer and the dance.
>
> I see the ways to be completely absorbed in the details of my performance.

_____

_____

_____

## D.  APPLICATION OF ANCIENT WISDOM

Use the following pragmatic shifts in attitude to help restructure your conceptual view of the world around you:

> *Review the philosophical tenets of Tao, especially in the dance of the Yin-Yang polarity of Tai Ji. Concentrate on feeling the Qi*

*flowing throughout your entire body, spontaneously, unclut-*
*tered, without tension and too much thought. Enjoy the race*
*and flowing exhilaration of Feng Liu (windflow). Remember, Na-*
*ture is the Dance!*

YEH

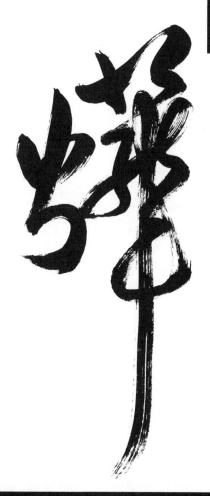

A blaze of fire
The splendor of flowers in full bloom

*I*n this, the second stage of your physio-spiritual journey, you begin to learn how subtle shifts in consciousness can encourage you to move ahead with our physical agenda in a healthier emotional and internally dynamic way. It is here that you will discover the sense of personal passion, acceptance and deep commitment to the daily process of working out as well as working within. You will begin to understand that not to take personal risks in life is, indeed, the greatest risk of all. Rather than follow blindly the "no pain, no gain" philosophy, you will see how you can gain without strain, not only in sports and exercise but in all of life. To overcome your inertia towards exercise, you will experience the way to project your Qi, your life's energy force, for the resurgence of energy when needed. Finally, for all of us who have difficulty delaying gratification, apply the ancient Chinese paradox: go slower, arrive sooner. As with every stage on this journey, you will be encouraged to focus on the pure spirit of play, a magic place where you have the opportunity to use your physical work to cultivate deep inner fitness.

# Power of Passion

Every day, when he arrived home from work, he would join the kids in the neighborhood for an exciting game of stickball. The sewers were the bases and broomsticks were the bats; they would play for hours until it was too dark to see the ball. He played with fire in his eyes and passion in his heart, igniting within each player the spirit of enthusiasm. He had the power of love for his sport, that magic ingredient that enables each of us to get beyond the obstacles and barriers blocking our full potential. His play on the streets of New York City was passionate, the same love he brought to his job as center fielder for the then New York Giants. He was one of the greatest, most passionate athletes ever to play the game of baseball. His name: Willie Mays. He loved what he did and instilled that love in all who played with him, young and old. He had achieved a goal that few ever consider possible: to create a marriage between avocation and vocation. Imagine getting paid for doing something you'd be doing anyway, even it you weren't paid for it.

To follow the Tao is to follow the way of passion. It is the way life was meant to be lived. Tapping into this magic potion is an important aspect of the joy, fulfillment and success in any of life's endeavors. To experience it in sports and exercise helps you to feel its power and encourages you to search for it in other arenas of life.

First, begin to search for a sport or physical program that fits snugly over your spirit (assuming you haven't done so thus far). By this we mean to choose activities that coincide with your skills, talents, and, above all, passion, or what you intuitively feel is best for you; this will help to guide you past your initial fears, failures, setbacks and anxieties along the way. It will help you to rise to the top rather than to fight your way there. Such choices will enable you to remain motivated and sustain your interest in the physical; without the passionate connection, exercise, working out and sports could always be a struggle for you.

Not that there won't be struggle with the path of passion. It's just that through passion, you will be better equipped to hurdle the barriers. A world-class river kayaker talks about the river as a metaphor for the inner journey of passion in all of life:

> You must love the river and all of its personalities; it constantly changes direction and, at times, seems to be going back to the start. The pace quickens rapidly through the narrows yet dramatically slows as the river widens. Sometimes the water is clear, sometimes murky and cloudy; exhilarating yet placid; raging yet calm. If you try to slow down when it speeds up, you struggle; if you speed up when it slows down, it will resist. You can't push the river.

Paddle upstream and frustration will take over. You can choose to end the trip at any time, but you will do so at your own risk. To experience a most exuberant journey, give yourself over to the power of the river, and feel the spiritual aspects of what it has to offer. If you could see the river's path (your inner journey) from a higher perspective, you would see clearly that there is a natural progression and flow, a journey with ups and downs, turns and surprises, cloudy and clear times. Let it flow! You need to trust—it's a must if you are to experience a deep sense of passion in life.

Notice how you get turned on when you begin to choose activities worth playing and doing for yourself. A labor of love is extremely rewarding, no matter how long it takes to master. Apply this same principle with any endeavor in life. When you choose what you love, be it work, relationships or places to live, all will come easier to you and the satisfaction will be exponential.

Once you identify a passion, let it burn inside until it consumes you. When you do, notice how spiritually alive you feel. You begin to tingle as you experience a sense of accomplishment and freedom. When you do, your life (and physical world) will change forever. It's comforting to look back upon your years and notice that the best of times, when you felt good about yourself, were the moments when you have been on target with your heart, your passion and what you loved. These were the times when your soul and spirit felt elevated. The way to experience this connection is to get in touch with who you are and what you really want in life. Ask yourself what you truly value and then create a marriage between what you value and the activity you choose. Next, ask yourself what activity in sports, exercise or life you would choose if success were guaranteed? Your answer probably indicates a passion for that particular game, event or activity. Follow your heart, and passion will be yours for a lifetime.

Use the following exercises to help you gain the power of passion. Remember, also, that you will want to precede your daily workout or sports activity with a ten-minute Tao Mind breathing and visualization session to help you relax and focus on how you wish to perform your exercise regimen:

## A.  BREATH WATCHING

Again, in our relaxed Tao Mind state, with eyes closed:

- Inhale slowly through nostrils and watch with your eyes closed the "white cloud" fill the lungs completely.

- Suspend breath for a few seconds (three to five) and watch the clean air travel to all extremities of your body.

- Exhale and watch the "smoky de-oxygenated cloud" exit the nostrils as carbon dioxide. See it dissolve and disappear.

- Suspend breath for a few seconds (three to five) and imagine the emptiness of your lungs.

- Repeat this breath-watching process ten or more times and notice the calm relaxation take over.

## B.  VISUALIZATION

Again, in your relaxed Tao Mind state, with eyes closed:

- *Tell* yourself all the reasons why your physical activity thrills and excites you.

- *Feel* the joy that it creates, knowing this is the reason you do it.

- *Be consumed* by your passion as you keep the excitement going.

- *Feel* deep within, those feelings you had when you initially began to participate.

- *Sense* the exhilaration that accompanies the passion you experience.

- *Play* your game in the spirit of love, free of judgment or criticism.

## C.  AFFIRMATIONS

Remember that the following are samples of affirmations that reinforce the Tao lesson to be learned. On the blank lines provided, create some affirmations that are more personal and relevant to your journey. Experiment and have fun in the process and make good use of index cards, posting your affirmations in a variety of places. Also recite them to yourself during visualization and picture what the words actually say.

When I do what I love, I love what I do.

I ignite the fire of my spirit to suit my body.

I follow my heart and that's the best part.

_____

_____

_____

## D. APPLICATION OF ANCIENT WISDOM

Use the following pragmatic shifts in attitude to help restructure your conceptual view of the world around you:

> *Fire is the key to your passion. Pay attention to the area of your lower abdomen (Dantien-hara), the gut belly feeling within. Identify a small warm flame inside, ignite it with a "HA!" sound. Feel it ablaze, filling your body with Fire energy as you stand up tall. Place both hands in front of your belly with your palms feeling the heat. Inhale deeply and fully; release your breath as you step forward and shout "Hwoo-awe" with joy as you fling your arms up, waving over your head. Imagine and identify your body as a glowing flame, burning bright, your inner light shining.*

# Acceptance Is Action

According to the *Tao Te Ching*, people who are accepting will ascend; those who are not will descend. A peaceful, accepting frame of mind enables you to adjust to the existing circumstances with success. Resistance to change or the way things are causes hardness, tension, anxiety and stress, all of which obstruct your potential. Rigid tree branches break in a storm; Chinese bamboo bends softly and bounces back unharmed.

Learning acceptance is not easy for anyone. It is a form of self-realization, a huge leap of faith enabling you to come to terms with the way things are, not the way you think they should be. By their very unpredictable nature, sports and exercise are divine teachers affording you the opportunity to test your levels of frustration when circumstances or events change rapidly without warning. For example, many athletes are well prepared and trained, yet they do not live up to their billing. A national-class cyclist, competing in the Olympic trials, talked about feeling helpless as she was struggling with an "off day" during this important event. "How can I accept that?" she asked. To fight the reality is to further the struggle.

Which she did. Her anger and fury over the helpless situation further hampered her efforts. When you find yourself having an "off day" in any arena of performance, it is better to accept the situation, relax and ask yourself: "Since I'm having an off day, what *can* I do now; what am I able to do if I can't do it all?" By asking these questions, you take positive action by doing what is possible and you reduce the stress and anxiety associated with trying to come to terms with the struggle. When things fail to go your way, acceptance and adaptation will help you to function at higher levels and feel better internally during the process.

Many of us also have difficulty accepting injury or illness. Such setbacks halt your physical efforts instantly. Yet, here is where sports and exercise offer the perfect opportunity for inner growth if you choose to use this downtime for reflection and meditation, a time to examine your training program, to ask sacred questions, such as "Where am I? Where am I going? Could I do things better? Am I happy with what I'm doing?" Here is a situation that truly tests what you are made of, whether or not you are flexible enough to go with the flow.

Yet it's easy to resist acceptance. You may fear that it is synonymous with resignation, a state of predestination where action is useless. Nothing could be further from the truth. Acceptance is truly a sign that you are in tune with a given situation and, knowing who you really are, take positive steps that will help you to optimize your potential. It often means the difference between success or failure. Acceptance is a definite soulful choice, a deeply spiritual act taking you beyond a state of inertness. Accepting "what is" shows an inner strength, one that requires you to assess the situation thoroughly, ascertain what is required in order to function adequately, adapt and then act accordingly. For example, people who inhabit desert regions are not fatalistic about plant life. Given a dry, hot climate, they don't plant flowers that need lots of water; they accept the environment and plant succulents. Accept—adapt—act. It is the action that steers you away from helplessness.

Acceptance of their environment proved to be beneficial for the UCLA basketball program. For the fourteen years prior to their first of ten national collegiate championships, the Bruins had no real home court, playing their games at a variety of local venues. According to their coach, John Wooden, this adversity became a considerable advantage as they became more comfortable on "foreign" turf. Acceptance of their situation helped turn adversity into opportunity.

As you begin to get physically fit and well conditioned, you need to assess the present shape you are in and accept this openly. Once you do accept your physical state, get down to the business of taking appropriate action. Remember that as you take an inventory of what you lack, consider what you have going for you and be sure to emphasize those qualities (physical, mental, spiritual traits) that will help to encourage you and ignite the fires of physical resurgence.

Once you learn the Tao lesson of acceptance in sports and exercise, you are ready to apply it to all of life. The key is to emphasize what you have by letting it keep you afloat during the early stages of self-development rather than focus totally on what you lack. You may not be the best speaker or the most knowledgeable teacher at this time, but your innate charisma, charm and caring nature will keep you going until you develop these skills. Notice and nurture what you do have and you will begin to develop that which you don't. Basically, you need to have the grace and wisdom to accept the aspects of self that you cannot change and to alter those you can. A true champion in sport as well as a winner in life does not have it all. One may only use what one does have—repeatedly—and use it well.

Use the following exercises to help you cultivate inner talent and to nurture and reinforce the concept of acceptance. Remember, also, that you will want to precede your daily workout or sports activity with a ten-minute Tao Mind breathing and visualization session to help you relax and focus on how you wish to perform your exercise regimen:

## A.  BREATH WATCHING

Again, in our relaxed Tao Mind state, with eyes closed:

- Inhale slowly through nostrils and watch with your eyes closed the "white cloud" fill the lungs completely.

- Suspend breath for a few seconds (three to five) and watch the clean air travel to all extremities of your body.

- Exhale and watch the "smoky de-oxygenated cloud" exit the nostrils as carbon dioxide. See it dissolve and disappear.

- Suspend breath for a few seconds (three to five) and imagine the emptiness of your lungs.

- Repeat this breath-watching process ten or more times and notice the calm relaxation take over.

## B.  VISUALIZATION

Again, in your relaxed Tao Mind state, with eyes closed:

- *Notice* all your positive physical qualities.

- *See* them in action as you perform.

- *Notice* your shortcomings.

- *Accept* them for what they are.

- *Feel* yourself adjusting and relying on all your strengths to pull you through.

- *See* yourself doing quite well under the circumstances.

- *Feel* your strength through acceptance as you refuse to stagnate.

## C.  AFFIRMATIONS

Remember that the following are samples of affirmations that reinforce the Tao lesson to be learned. On the blank lines provided, create some affirmations that are more personal and relevant to your journey. Experiment and have fun in the process and make good use of index cards, posting your affirmations in a variety of places.

Also recite them to yourself during visualization and picture what the words actually say.

I accept, so I can adjust, assess, adapt and *act.*

I lack, therefore I add and I advance.

I am perfectly happy the way I am.

_____

_____

_____

## D.  APPLICATION OF ANCIENT WISDOM

Use the following pragmatic shifts in attitude to help restructure your conceptual view of the world around you:

*Water is the Tao metaphor to be experienced here. Sit and relax for a few moments before and after each workout. Feel the flowing water element throughout your entire body as it becomes supple and flexible as water. Your blood is circulating through clear canals without obstruction. Reach upward and overhead with your arms and scoop the flowing Water Qi back into the body. Feel the cascading sensation entering the entire body, from the crown of your head down the spine, through the buttocks, into the legs and feet, and continuing deep down into the ground. Feel totally regenerated, simply by accepting and receiving the Water force of life.*

# Making a Sacred Pledge

At this stage of the journey you want to be sure that your attempt at physical and inner fitness is a lifelong one. In order to have this happen, consider taking a pledge to commit and persevere. The *I Ching* is quick to remind us how all significant deeds are accomplished through an enduring effort in a consistent direction. It talks about how positive perseverance in all endeavors leads to good fortune. Take the pledge and you will attain full benefit from your program each day of your life.

Perseverance is not a pushy or forceful path. It requires that you relax and be patient as the situation gradually unfolds in your favor. You might as well take the time to enjoy the journey because there really is no destination; there is no place at which you arrive. Physical and inner fitness are never ending; they begin anew each day of your life. Accepting this, and understanding its relevancy for all of life is, in itself, a spiritual consciousness. When you persevere, you begin to notice all of the positive personal benefits along the way: You do get to the mountaintop; you do create a soulful book; you do manage to find work that nurtures the spirit; you do find a passionate, loving relationship.

It's simple yet, initially, not easy: Each day as you rise, you must commit yourself to the sacred virtue of perseverance, and seek out the ways in which you can accomplish this through sports and exercise. For example, there will be a time when you will be tormented by the demons of temptation to quit the match, the game or the program. Imagine you are playing tennis and you are down two sets and 5–love in the third and realize that few athletes ever make up such a huge deficit. However, you decide that giving up is no alternative. You dig down deep and choose to play with integrity. The palm trees are beginning to appear on the horizon, so to speak, and you persevere, one point at a time. You could make the comeback of your tennis career yet, regardless of your apparent success on the scoreboard, the greater victory will come from within. You learned never to lose heart and to persevere in every aspect of your life.

During this time of self-expansion, it is imperative that you commit to going the distance. Pledge to march ahead even during adversity. In thinking about perseverance and commitment, we know that when refinishing an antique table, the classic piece must suffer the pain of the tough sanding process, yet what emerges is something special. If any of us hopes to be special, we must persevere even when the going gets tough. Be willing to do all that's required to keep you rolling on this path. Persevering is, by itself, a conscious spiritual choice, a sacred pledge, to devote the necessary time and effort required to realize this dream of full-spectrum fitness. If your level of commitment each and every day is strong, your journey will be successful and much fun. Commitment to persevering reduces any hesitancy you may have, and forward movement will come naturally. The moment you commit, Providence, the benevolent guidance of nature, of the Tao, takes over. Your friends, acquaintances and the universe seem to conspire to enable you to realize your potential. In this way, the act of perseverance becomes a spiritual aphrodisiac, turning you on to and getting you stimulated for the working-out and working-within process.

Once again, sports and fitness are ideal arenas to test your ability to persevere. Remember that most of us start and stop a program of physical fitness on the average of thirteen times. With a slight shift in consciousness, your focus on fitness begins to widen and interest soars as these dynamic efforts become obvious. When you begin to experience the advantages of persevering with your physical program, you will discover its benefits in the rest of life. For example, it takes most of us a few years for our bodies to adjust to a higher level of activity. Through diligent training and perseverance, your body becomes able to handle greater amounts of exertion; it adapts readily to stress from the consistent, daily conditioning. Seeing this in the physical realm may teach you that consistency of effort is, indeed, rewarded. You may apply this lesson to your profession and personal life and discover similar results.

Perhaps we can remember the perseverance of people like superstar Michael Jordan. Told he wasn't good enough to play for his high school varsity basketball team, he worked diligently on his game every day and persevered until he proved his coach was wrong. Author Richard Bach had one of his best books rejected for publication eighty-two times; with perseverance, it became a bestseller. Albert Einstein, Jonas Salk and Thomas Edison made major contributions to this world all because they persevered, in spite of numerous setbacks.

At times, perseverance may seem difficult or problematic; when doubt appears and you begin to feel yourself waver on your pledge, use the various Tao lessons throughout this book to comfort you. When you fall away from your daily routine, simply begin again, a new beginning filled with hope and excitement. Know that the process of starting and stopping is a natural one; everyone experiences it. It is, perhaps, more important to remain in this process than try to reach the goal. You exhibit real success when you choose to focus on this process rather than the product and begin once again after you have stopped. That is *the* actual pledge: to continue amid adversity. During difficult periods along this journey, remember that setbacks are natural and you can choose to emerge from the setback. Therefore, stick with it and begin again each day to practice the sacred act of perseverance for the game of life.

Use the following exercises to help you cultivate perseverance. Remember, also, that you will want to precede your daily workout or sports activity with a ten-minute Tao Mind breathing and visualization session to help you relax and focus on how you wish to perform your exercise regimen:

## A. BREATH WATCHING

Again, in our relaxed Tao Mind state, with eyes closed:

- Inhale slowly through nostrils and watch with your eyes closed the "white cloud" fill the lungs completely.

- Suspend breath for a few seconds (three to five) and watch the clean air travel to all extremities of your body.

- Exhale and watch the "smoky de-oxygenated cloud" exit the nostrils as carbon dioxide. See it dissolve and disappear.

- Suspend breath for a few seconds (three to five) and imagine the emptiness of your lungs.

- Repeat this breath-watching process ten or more times and notice the calm relaxation take over.

## B. VISUALIZATION

Again, in your relaxed Tao Mind state, with eyes closed:

- *Pledge* to yourself: "I am totally committed to a path of spiritual fitness for life."

- *Feel* healthy, vibrant and open to learning life's lessons through physical activity.

- *See* yourself get off track for a while and, when you do,

- *Recite* once again, your pledge and begin, once again, to follow the path.

- *Feel* the satisfaction that comes from staying connected to your commitment.

## C. AFFIRMATIONS

Remember that the following are samples of affirmations that reinforce the Tao lesson to be learned. On the blank lines provided, create some affirmations that are more personal and relevant to your journey. Experiment and have fun in the process and make good use of index cards, posting your affirmations in a variety of places. Also recite them to yourself during visualization and picture what the words actually say.

I begin each day, in a new way, to pledge to play.

My commitment is to continue the best I can.

I simply say: "Yes, I can" and "Yes, I will."

_____

_____

_____

## D. APPLICATION OF ANCIENT WISDOM

Use the following pragmatic shifts in attitude to help restructure your conceptual view of the world around you:

*Believe in the power of Qi, and the constancy of Change and Transformation of I (yee). Gather in all the power deep down in your Dantien-belly. Extend your arms and legs wide to get in touch with all the changing and swirling energy around you. Pull back your arms into the center of your body, and shout "Yes" and "Ha." Do it several times, as you make your pledge to honor and submit to the true power inside your physical body. Feel wonderful and strong with your fortified Dantien center. Smile, and carry on with your sport or workout routine.*

# The Risk of Not Risking

Charlie had been a successful dentist for many years, but began to feel the pangs of remorse setting in. He would always wonder what life would have been like had he chosen golf as his vocation. When he would share this dream with close personal friends, they would dismiss it as childish nonsense, impossible and foolhardy. With love and encouragement from his wife, Charlie decided to quit his practice, follow his passion and take to the road to see if he could qualify for the Professional Golf Association tour. He was determined to devote one year of his life to find out if he had the skill and ability to play at that level. Charlie didn't do as well as he thought he could; he was sad but relieved. When a friend of his asked how he could have taken such a foolish risk, Charlie commented how disappointing it would have been to *not* have taken the risk, to have lived with the remorse and regret of not having tried and always wondering "What if . . . ?" He awakened the spiritual in this friend with this statement of wisdom.

The risk of not risking, what Charlie faced, is something many of us confront in our lifetime. So much in life goes unexplored because we lack the courage to take the risk to follow our dreams in the face of potential failure. To not take the risk is, indeed, the greatest risk of all.

The wisdom of Tao regards risks as nature's way of making you inwardly courageous and strong. They are part of being alive, ushering in new meaning, richness and a deep awareness of life. The Chinese describe risk as thrill and adventure, an out-of-body-into-death experience that gives you the chance to be reborn into a new life.

A new life was what Christie, a female professional mountain biker, had coming to her. Short on confidence in the pro circuit, but tall on spirit, she demonstrated how taking a risk can create a positive shift in attitude. Many athletes in the world of cycling are familiar with the ever-so-famous wide and risky "water jump crossing" in Michigan. When she initially came upon it, she thought, "Next year." Yet, feeling down from a discouraging season, she decided that success here would give her an emotional lift and boost in confidence. Following ten minutes of visualization in the Tao Mind state, she rode to the top of the hill, put the bike in her biggest gear, raced down with courage and cleanly cleared the jump. Having the courage to risk paid off, giving her renewed belief in herself as an athlete and as a person. The word *courage* is related to the French *coeur*, which means "heart." In Chinese, the word for courage also means to dare. Christie dared to follow her heart, what she intuitively knew she needed. In this sense, her bike risk-taking became a sacred act of trusting and acting according to the Tao, her inner natural truth, what she knew to be right. Sports and exercise present numerous opportunities to take a risk and expand internally.

Like perseverance, risks are spiritual aphrodisiacs turning you on to life, instilling in those who dare stimulation, excitement, motivation and a deep sense of being fully alive. Having said this, it's equally crucial to understand that the "high" is in the process itself. Success, like everything else on this journey, is measured by the dance. The dance is filled with truths and lessons that make for a wider, if not longer, life. It's important not to measure self-esteem by an outcome or result once you take the risk.

Taking risks in cycling and running throughout my athletic life has taught me (Jerry) the importance of trusting and following my heart. I learned many years ago that the act of trusting is a higher state than that of doubting. Although it's easier to doubt, trusting is much more spiritually rewarding. Disgruntled with my situation in California, I decided to search for the Holy Grail and find Nirvana elsewhere. After a few years of research, my family and I followed my dream and chose beautiful Colorado as our new home. It wasn't easy to leave our work, friends and family behind, along with a community that was the spine for our support system for seventeen years. After six months in our beautiful newly built home in the foothills on the eastern slope of the Rockies, we realized that our biggest fear had come true; we missed our true home in Santa Cruz. It took a lot of courage to make the move to Colorado, but even more to trust these new feelings. When we look back on this experience, our loss on paper was exponentially overshadowed by the gains on a deeper, more spiritual level. Taking this risk brought the family closer together, gave my kids a better sense about themselves, and my wife, Jan, a whole new perspective on her confidence in business. More than all this, however, was the inner peace and certainty I gained from knowing exactly where I want to live. Had we not trusted the path of heart, we would still be spiritually unrested, always wondering why the grass always seems to be greener someplace else. Sometimes in life, you have to take a huge risky trip to discover that the treasure that you're searching for is right under the oak tree in your front yard. Taking such a trip is very expensive, but nothing compared to the cost of mental health.

During your physio-sacred journey, you will be presented with many opportunities to take risks and to trust that they can lead to potential openings and breakthroughs in sports and life. You may get hurt from time to time when you trust, but to not do so could lead to a life of torment. When risks arise, assess their importance to you and be willing to leave the dock, set sail and go off to sea. Taking a risk may seem threatening and scary, but you need to weigh the pain of taking the risk against the potential pain of not trying. Provided it is not life threatening, you need to consider the options involved and refuse to let self-doubt stand in your way. Let your physical risks strengthen you internally, making you inwardly fit to risk changing professions, moving your home, going back to school or any other risks that, from time to time, stare you in the face. If you feel trapped and lack the courage to take the risk, think about past risks taken that worked out successfully. What was your initial fear and did it materialize? How did you feel once you took the risk? Is it not a bigger risk to not risk? Answers to these questions can be the impetus you need to begin and trust the process of risk-taking. When you do, simply do your best and assume that all will work out as it should. Feel the exhilaration from your decision to feel alive.

Use the following exercises to help you cultivate inner talent and to nurture and reinforce taking risks. Remember, also, that you will want to precede your daily workout or sports activity with a ten-minute Tao Mind breathing and visualization session to help you relax and focus on how you wish to perform your exercise regimen:

## A. BREATH WATCHING

Again, in our relaxed Tao Mind state, with eyes closed:

- Inhale slowly through nostrils and watch with your eyes closed the "white cloud" fill the lungs completely.

- Suspend breath for a few seconds (three to five) and watch the clean air travel to all extremities of your body.

- Exhale and watch the "smoky de-oxygenated cloud" exit the nostrils as carbon dioxide. See it dissolve and disappear.

- Suspend breath for a few seconds (three to five) and imagine the emptiness of your lungs.

- Repeat this breath-watching process ten or more times and notice the calm relaxation take over.

## B. VISUALIZATION

Again, in your relaxed Tao Mind state, with eyes closed:

- *Imagine* taking a risk that you've been wanting to take.

- *Feel* your nervous tension and anxiety, common feelings when taking a risk.

- *Feel* yourself begin to relax and be calm as you begin to perform.

- *Hear* the voices of others give you praise for taking the chance.

- *Feel* very satisfied for having such courage to risk.

- *Open* your heart to learning from the experience.

- *Celebrate!*

## C. AFFIRMATIONS

Remember that the following are samples of affirmations that reinforce the Tao lesson to be learned. On the blank lines provided, create some affirmations that are more personal and relevant to your journey. Experiment and have fun in the process and make good use of index cards, posting your affirmations in a variety of places. Also recite them to yourself during visualization and picture what the words actually say.

I come alive when I take risks.

I feel the warrior spirit as I forge ahead.

I know I succeed when I try.

I am capable and ready to create my own affirmation. I do it now.

_____

_____

_____

## D. APPLICATION OF ANCIENT WISDOM

Use the following pragmatic shifts in attitude to help restructure your conceptual view of the world around you:

> *First settle back into a safe and secure stance. Relax for a moment. Do nothing. Now, suddenly, take a few steps forward, then a few back, a couple to the left, then right. Find out how you feel about these new placements of being where and who you are. How are you doing? Don't you feel excited with energizing adrenaline flowing? In Tai Ji work, centering is only meaningful when you can redefine it as you constantly make adjustment to change. Enjoy the notion of Crisis in Chinese, as both "danger" and "opportunity." Take the risk. Jump into another dimension—be surprised!*

# Project Your Qi

The Tao teaches how life is a constantly changing and growing process that takes place amid the Qi energies that circulate throughout all matter. The space that exists between the heavens and the earth, according to ancient wisdom, is filled with Qi. Chinese artists, through the great sweeping curves of their calligraphy, show the flowing movement of Qi, the streams of energy through nature.

In Chinese, your Qi is that deep, dynamic, spiritual life force or energy that you experience when mind and body are in sync. It is an inner strength that is impossible to see and difficult to explain, but, like most concepts of Tao, it can be experienced. For example, ask a friend to face you ten feet away and extend his or her arm firmly straight out to the side. Walk toward and into that arm. Now do this again and, as you do, look to a point beyond the extended arm and walk "through" it to that distant point. Notice the difference the second time when you project your Qi, your energy, forward.

All exercise stimulates the flow of Qi, thus creating a solid bond between these two physical and spiritual forces. You can notice how revitalized people's spirits become doing yoga, dance or the Chinese movement art of Tai Ji. Breath watching, one of the techniques used in this book for cultivating your inner talent, restores your Qi as well. The word for breath in Latin is *spiritus*. When you breath in, you inspire—take in the spirit and feel the inspiration, the energy to be creative. If you write or paint, for example, practice deep breathing prior to your efforts, and you will enhance and stimulate the flow of your creative juices.

In sports and fitness programs, Qi regulation and projection can be quite an asset. Projecting your energy into a game or workout is an important component of being fully present in body, mind and spirit for that activity. When athletes are standing on the sideline, they usually have difficulty performing when abruptly called off the bench. It takes awhile for their level of excitement to match the flow of the contest. This is similar to how demanding it is to begin a workout if you have been sitting behind a desk or in a car for hours. Changing gears is not easy. However, you can learn through the use of visualization to project your Qi into places outside your body, particularly into an arena of performance prior to entering. Depending upon what the mind sees, whether it's energy or fatigue, the central nervous system accepts it as if that state were real.

Athletes from the University of Maryland NCAA championship women's lacrosse team asked me (Jerry) how they could overcome the lull of standing on the sideline, so that when called upon to perform, they could raise their energy level to match that of the players already in the flow of the game. For these athletes, I asked them to breathe deeply and visualize themselves in the game with their full spirit, moving around in their position, doing what they'd do if called into action now. They were asked to imagine the adrenaline, the rush, excitement and movement as if they were actually playing. Those who followed my suggestions experienced the transition from standing around to playing with intensity as smooth and instantaneous as if they had been playing all along because when they mentally projected their Qi their adrenaline began to flow. Their nervous systems interpreted their visions to be real and this signaled the adrenal glands to respond accordingly. When you project your Qi through this imagery process, you cue the synchronization of millions of neural and muscular events necessary to make this experience possible.

The same applies to you and your fitness routines that require a sudden burst of energy. For example, driving in your car to the spa or gym is energy draining. In order to get into the workout groove, project your Qi as you drive. Visualize, in a Tao Mind state, all the joy and exhilaration you experience during exercise. Through ten or more deep breaths, feel relaxed and ready to immerse your spirit, that playful child, into your exercise regime. Follow the Tao by honoring your own pulse, rhythms, feelings and your own inner dance. Begin to sense the transition from sitting in the car to working out with intensity.

This can also be used if you're out for a run and getting to the top of a hill seems prohibitive; disassociate from the goal and focus instead on the energy you have to simply run and enjoy the smells and sounds of nature. Before you know it you'll be at the top.

Environment is an important component of Qi as well. During the Olympics in Atlanta, American athletes related how they received an extra boost from the boisterous fans. Carl Lewis, gold medalist in the long jump, talked about how he was on the brink of elimination when the roar of the crowd gave him what he needed to win his event. Other athletes claimed that, had it not been for the spirit of the "hometown" spectators, they may not have won gold. They experienced the Qi of a well-chosen nurturing environment. Make efforts to conduct your workout, if you can, in environments that will encourage and validate your activity. Exercise with others who will nudge you along. "Perform" your routine with the audience in the gym or spa. Or be alone in nature and absorb the spirit of that environment.

The same applies to all of life. Both of us live near the ocean part of the year, which provides energy from the waves and the salty taste of the sea. When Jerry lived in the mountains, he gathered strength from the massive rock formations. For Chungliang, Midwest farmland provides glorious sunrises and sunsets with great Qi power. For all of us, anywhere, use your visualization skills to great advantage by letting it stimulate your nervous system. For example, feel Qi power when you imagine being underneath a cascading waterfall as it pours energy into your entire body. Listen to its roaring sound, and enjoy the cleansing downpour and the sweet, stinging sensation upon your skin.

Now, for a burst of energy, try the following exercise:

*Stand up, extend your arms toward the sky and visualize your Qi flowing beyond your fingertips, and allow external (more powerful) Qi to enter your hands, through the fingers (with relaxed joints) and the spaces between fingers. Actively take five deep breaths and stretch (extend); passively exhale (release) and collect and receive Qi from beyond. See yourself gradually rise above the mundane routine exercises of stretching the body and take on new emotional and spiritual dimensions. Feel elated and filled up with plenty of positive and exhilarating Qi power of life.*

Use the following exercises to help you cultivate inner talent and to nurture and reinforce projecting your Qi. Remember, also, that you will want to precede your daily workout or sports activity with a ten-minute Tao Mind breathing and visualization session to help you relax and focus on how you wish to perform your exercise regimen:

## A. BREATH WATCHING

Again, in our relaxed Tao Mind state, with eyes closed:

- Inhale slowly through nostrils and watch with your eyes closed the "white cloud" fill the lungs completely.

- Suspend breath for a few seconds (three to five) and watch the clean air travel to all extremities of your body.

- Exhale and watch the "smoky de-oxygenated cloud" exit the nostrils as carbon dioxide. See it dissolve and disappear.

- Suspend breath for a few seconds (three to five) and imagine the emptiness of your lungs.

- Repeat this breath-watching process ten or more times and notice the calm relaxation take over.

## B. VISUALIZATION

Again, in your relaxed Tao Mind state, with eyes closed:

- *Choose* a sports or exercise to participate in with high energy.

- *Feel* yourself performing with ease and agility.

- *Sense* the adrenaline as it pumps through your body.

- *Feel* excited and energized as you fill up with exhilarating Qi power.

## C. AFFIRMATIONS

Remember that the following are samples of affirmations that reinforce the Tao lesson to be learned. On the blank lines provided, create some affirmations that are more personal and relevant to your journey. Experiment and have fun in the process and make good use of index cards, posting your affirmations in a variety of places. Also recite them to yourself during visualization and picture what the words actually say.

I absorb an abundance of positive energy from my total environment.

I send my feelers and receptacles to tap and receive all the positive, energizing Qi around me.

_____

_____

_____

## D. APPLICATION OF ANCIENT WISDOM

Use the following pragmatic shifts in attitude to help restructure
your conceptual view of the world around you:

*Once again, test your projection of Qi. Close your eyes and feel
the inner light and warmth deep inside and the power all around
you. Set your "pilot light" aflame. Ignite your passion. "Follow
the Force!"*

# Go Slower,
# Arrive Sooner

Tao wisdom encourages a calm observation of the natural unfolding of events. Rapid growth and advancement are unnatural. One's potential blossoms in a gradual way. Therefore, it is wise to avoid haste and enjoy the moment as you come into your own. Taoist philosopher Lao Tzu encourages patience and reminds us how all things occur at the appropriate time. Patience is the ability to enjoy and immerse yourself in the process, the flow of life, as it assumes its own form and shape.

An athlete went to her coach and asked how long it would take to develop into a world-class triathlete. He reassured her that if she trained properly, it would take four to five years to come into her own. Feeling frustrated and uneasy about this, she told him she didn't want to wait that long. In an attempt to force the issue and arrive on the scene sooner, she asked how long it would take if she worked harder, faster and with more effort. Ten to twelve years was his reply.

You are about to enter into a new time zone where slowing down is faster than speeding up. Sports and exercise create numerous opportunities for you to slow down, develop and practice the sacred virtue of patience. We recommend that you develop strength in this area through "Wait Training": Notice the natural flow of events and then act accordingly. This requires constant vigilance as you monitor your progress with regard to levels of energy, fatigue, soreness, staleness, slumps, plateaus, spurts, enthusiasm and burn-out. Too much, too soon, that familiar "hurry-up" sickness, invariably leads to injury or illness, nature's way of telling you to slow down, reevaluate and take a break.

When you restart your exercise or sports program, know that it will take time to develop your body and the capacity to endure the physical demands placed upon it. Refuse to get trapped by comparing your progress to others. When snags and obstacles do come your way, don't fight them or get too discouraged. Accept and acknowledge these setbacks as opportunities to learn while you physically emerge. With patience, you will find openings, solutions, and resolutions. Try to rush and you'll be greeted by tension, anxiety and an ultimate "delay of game" penalty; slower is indeed quicker.

It's important that you don't think of patience as the capacity to endure, or as an act of perseverance. See it, instead, as the willingness to be at peace and give yourself time to work toward your goal without placing limits on how long it will take to reach it. Patience is a mind-set that goes beyond the connotation of suffering. This is not about pain in any way. Remember that in sports, as in all of life, things occur not when we think they should but when the time is right. According to the Tao, there is a natural flow to all events; chaos results when you try to hasten the natural process.

Experiencing the immediate effects of patience, or lack of same, in your physical arena should make it easier to apply your wisdom in other aspects of life. On your trip across town you feel frustrated, annoyed and angry when every stoplight turns red as you approach the intersection. If you hurry up, you risk having an accident or being stopped by the police for going through a red light. You'll get to your destination more quickly and safely if you see each stop along the way as an opportune moment to meditate, reflect upon what's right in your life, take a few deep breaths, change the music or simply feel the peace of detaching yourself from the chaos of the outside world.

Patience is also a virtue that can help you when waiting for your plane to take off at the airport. It may be delayed because a mechanical problem needs to be resolved. Ultimately, your wait is rewarded by a safe arrival. Another plane, in an attempt to keep on schedule, overlooks safety requirements and runs the risk of never arriving. Slow down and get to where you're going sooner, and safer.

Think for a moment about the race between the tortoise and the hare. Through the inner spiritual qualities of consistent, deliberate, steady, slow movement, the tortoise arrives sooner than the quicker yet more spastic, inconsistent and fatigued hare. Haste, does, indeed, make waste.

Use the following exercises to help you cultivate inner talent and to nurture and reinforce the power of patience. Remember, also, that you will want to precede your daily workout or sports activity with a ten-minute Tao Mind breathing and visualization session to help you relax and focus on how you wish to perform your exercise regimen:

## A. BREATH WATCHING

Again, in our relaxed Tao Mind state, with eyes closed:

- Inhale slowly through nostrils and watch with your eyes closed the "white cloud" fill the lungs completely.

- Suspend breath for a few seconds (three to five) and watch the clean air travel to all extremities of your body.

- Exhale and watch the "smoky de-oxygenated cloud" exit the nostrils as carbon dioxide. See it dissolve and disappear.

- Suspend breath for a few seconds (three to five) and imagine the emptiness of your lungs.

- Repeat this breath-watching process ten or more times and notice the calm relaxation take over.

## B. VISUALIZATION

Again, in your relaxed Tao Mind state, with eyes closed:

- *Think* of an event or a task that causes you to be impatient.

- *See* yourself performing in a hurried-up manner, making mistakes and getting upset.

- *Accept* these setbacks as warnings for you to slow down.

- *Relax*, be at peace and begin to take your time without limiting yourself.

- *Feel* yourself flow with the task as you perform excellently and more efficiently.

## C. AFFIRMATIONS

Remember that the following are samples of affirmations that reinforce the Tao lesson to be learned. On the blank lines provided, create some affirmations that are more personal and relevant to your journey. Experiment and have fun in the process and make good use of index cards, posting your affirmations in a variety of places. Also recite them to yourself during visualization and picture what the words actually say.

My patience is the virtue of my success.

When I slow down, I get into the flow and get there in the perfect time.

I know: "Well done is soon enough!"

_____

_____

_____

## D.  APPLICATION OF ANCIENT WISDOM

Use the following pragmatic shifts in attitude to help restructure your conceptual view of the world around you:

> Tai Ji practice is never in a rush to get someplace in the future. It is always in the present with the focus on the process. To experience this, wave your arms around the body slowly, feeling every detail of the joints throughout your arms, clicking into action, softly propelling the rippling and curvaceous motion. We call this powerful, graceful motion "Cloud Hands." As you enjoy this Tai Ji way of waving your arms, you'll find yourself slowing down, to savor this delicious and fun experience. You now have arrived at the place where you always want to be.

D J U

Uplifting high above
Centering and ascending within

*T*he *Tao Te Ching* teaches that every one of us possesses an incredible power or potential that is constantly available when we become aware of and align ourselves with the flow of nature, the way that things happen, a way that is beyond our control. If we notice how these forces work, and act in concert with them, life can be quite fulfilling. However, the price we pay for trying to control, fight or resist these natural patterns is a life full of limitations. Rubbing your hand vigorously against the grain on a slab of redwood could ruin your afternoon. Slicing turkey breast against the grain creates an aesthetic disaster. Fighting the ocean current can be exhausting and futile. As a matter of fact, Nature demands that you always go with the flow in anything you encounter; if we fail to act accordingly, problems ensue. For example, at birth, we are all in harmony with these natural patterns, created in a state of unlimited potential. Then, through years of exposure to society's limited beliefs, fears and attitudes, we become misaligned with the grand plan. We become conditioned to believe that there are certain limits to what we can or can't do, and as you know, people who believe in limits are limited people. The Tao tells us that when you align with the way of nature, the unlimited way, you experience your own greatness and fulfillment.

During the third stage of your Working Out, Working Within journey, you enter the compelling space of possibility and go beyond what you once thought were limits. Whether you decide to compete with others or with yourself, you will have ample opportunity to test your limitations by using your developing body and level of skills in your arena of choice. It is during this stage that you will learn how to open to your greatness and dispel the myths and attitudes of limitation. Following the opening chapter on Limitless Limits, you will learn how to understand and strengthen your confidence and how to nurture the wisdom of moderation and non-excessiveness. Next, you will encounter the concept of goals in a very different way, as they simply become lanterns that guide you along a path. Then, in order to progress along that unlimited path, you will examine your images of self, images that will nurture and support your journey of possibility. Finally, you will want to know the key to mastery in all that you do. It's simple, but not easy.

There is an inspirational story about unlimited possibility that will set the tone for the chapters within. It takes place in the mountains east of Los Angeles, at Big Bear. A runner became lost, cruising on trails at an elevation of nine thousand feet. As he approached a crossroads, he spotted three cyclists and decided to ask them for directions. They knew precisely how to exit the forest. Impressed with their knowledge of the terrain, the runner asked these athletes how often they rode this mountain. Said one, "We've been coming here five days a week for the past seven years. In the winter we ski. We first came on my birthday, when I turned seventy." His buddies were seventy-eight and seventy-five. Most people are somewhat shocked when they hear this story because they have preconceived ideas or limited beliefs about age and what you can or can't do at certain times of life. These three amigos teach us much about possibility.

By shifting your mental images and opening your mind to unlimited possibility, you can make a huge difference in your ability to see beyond what you thought were limits. If you consider the sky the limit, you will realize that, like the three cyclists in the above story, your upward stretch physically and mentally has, indeed, no limit. During your physical "workout," your sacred work "within" can grow tall and soar unlimitedly.

# Limitless Limits

Like the Tao, you are a natural process capable of continual growth and blossoming. In Confucian ethics, the unlimited person is one who constantly reassesses his or her state of being and is willing to do what it takes to improve. When you are in tune with the Tao, you possess the power of continual transformation, from being to becoming. According to Lao Tzu, this process of becoming requires you to be aware of your shortcomings and see yourself as a beginner, totally empty and ready to receive. When you think about it, the beginner has limitless possibilities; the expert has none.

Your power and strength in sports and exercise start with the deep humble sense that you are a beginner with unlimited potential, regardless of how much time you have devoted to your discipline. The concept of being totally empty and willing to learn is a precondition for unlimitedness. In Chinese, we call this empty place "Wu Ji," that which gives you the ability to face your insecurities and flow into the vast sea of potentiality, profound growth and improvement. With the Tao, we are reminded to travel openly on uncharted paths, remain empty and learn to sustain the Beginner's Mind.

Opening up to the unlimited boundaries of his vast potential was the choice of Keith Foreman. As a freshman "walk-on" on the University of Oregon men's track team, he was told how limited his possibilities were with an elite group of scholarship athletes. Yet Keith saw himself as a beginner with unlimited opportunity to learn, and he took on the challenge of competing with the best. He believed the sky was his only limit. Before he graduated, Keith became only the fifth American runner ever to break the four-minute mile barrier. Having accomplished this in sport, Keith seized the opportunity to grow spiritually and apply his confidence and strength to other endeavors in life. In his fifties, he continues to push the limitless boundaries of his potential, studying for an advanced doctoral degree and continuing to compete as a national-class athlete.

It's important to understand the difference between two types of limits. There are the "limiting limits," those that are actual, real obstacles defining the boundaries of your potential. For example, in basketball, your lack of height could be a real limiting factor in playing center for the Chicago Bulls; money will determine what you can or cannot afford to buy; without gas, your car won't go; humans can't fly. These are natural limits.

Then there are the "limitless limits," those that we *think* or *imagine* to be limits yet, with the right shift in consciousness, rarely become limiting factors. Most limitations fall into this category. It has been said that the average human being uses a mere fifteen percent of his or her physical and mental potential. We constantly underestimate our capabilities. We even are surrounded by global limited thinking. Consider this situation: After an in-depth study of the bumblebee, the world's best experts in the field of aerodynamics announced that the bee could not fly—it was too heavy, too slow, too small, and limited in numerous other ways. Fortunately, the bee couldn't read the final report. Unfortunately, we *can* hear and read, which often works to our disadvantage. Yet, when you refuse to listen, but instead you dig down deep and discover potentials through your physical activity that you never knew existed, you attain a level of spiritual growth that enables you to be open and receptive to what life has to offer when you say "yes" to all possibilities.

Many people have bought into stories of self-limitations. There are those who say we can't ski, we're too awkward, yet they see a talented skier with no legs; then they hear about the concert guitarist with no arms and reevaluate their limited thinking about playing music. People who argue for their limitations are limited. You need to know that, whatever you imagine your limitations in life to be, if you're willing to trust the enormous capacity for growth that you've been given and take the necessary steps to develop yourself, you will redefine and explore the boundaries of your full potential. The message of the *Tao Te Ching* is clear: Trust the power within and use it.

When faced with what you think are limitations, ask close friends for their input and watch your progress closely so you continue in the direction that contradicts these limits. Maybe they're real; maybe not. But at least you will have tried and discovered the truth.

Remember, too, that some limits can be useful, particularly in sports and physical activities. For example, you have a certain capacity when you begin to work out and it's good to not strain beyond in order to avoid injury. The same applies to life: You are able to take advantage of seeing a play or concert because you are aware that it's here for a limited time. Many signs of caution are limits that could save your life. For example, don't exceed the weight limitations for takeoff in a plane. It could prove costly.

Use the following exercises to help you cultivate a sense of limitless limits. Remember, also, that you will want to precede your daily workout or sports activity with a ten-minute Tao Mind breathing and visualization session to help you relax and focus on how you wish to perform your exercise regimen:

## A. BREATH WATCHING

Again, in our relaxed Tao Mind state, with eyes closed:

- Inhale slowly through nostrils and watch with your eyes closed the "white cloud" fill the lungs completely.

- Suspend breath for a few seconds (three to five) and watch the clean air travel to all extremities of your body.

- Exhale and watch the "smoky de-oxygenated cloud" exit the nostrils as carbon dioxide. See it dissolve and disappear.

- Suspend breath for a few seconds (three to five) and imagine the emptiness of your lungs.

- Repeat this breath-watching process ten or more times and notice the calm relaxation take over.

## B. VISUALIZATION

Again, in your relaxed Tao Mind state, with eyes closed:

- *Think* of a limit that you habitually place on yourself ("I'm too old, fat, slow, dumb," etc.).

- *See* yourself performing as if you are an athlete with great skill and dexterity.

- *Feel* in the grove, doing what you didn't think you could do.

- *Trust* that you have the necessary power to go beyond your limits.

- *Feel* the sensation and elation from beyond your limits.

## C. AFFIRMATIONS

Remember that the following are samples of affirmations that reinforce the Tao lesson to be learned. On the blank lines provided, create some affirmations that are more personal and relevant to your journey. Experiment and have fun in the process and make good use of index cards, posting your affirmations in a variety of places. Also recite them to yourself during visualization and picture what the words actually say.

I constantly redefine the limited boundaries of my full potential.

I see everything I have done as only the beginnings of unlimited change and transformation.

I can see the unlimited variations of my potentials unfolding in front of my eyes.

I see through the illusion of my limits. I am limitless.

_____

_____

_____

## D. APPLICATION OF ANCIENT WISDOM

Use the following pragmatic shifts in attitude to help restructure your conceptual view of the world around you:

*In Tao meditation, we come back fully into ourselves, body and soul. The small "me" is glaringly obvious. Within this contained being, we come into full power by projecting ourselves beyond and connecting with bigger and larger sources of life. Stand up. Stretch your arms and legs wide open. As you project your inner Qi out, you also funnel in the great power all around you. Be sure to focus your attention on your Dantien center, and trust your own power. This is your reality. This small body is unlimited indeed. Use it. It is inexhaustible.*

# Exhibiting a Presence

The University of Maryland women's lacrosse team, by defeating their opponents, the University of Virginia, won their second consecutive NCAA Division I championship. When the same two powerhouses met the following year in regular season play at UVA's home field, the emotional intensity was electric. It could have lit up a city. With Maryland down 4–3 at the half, their coach, Cindy Timchal, refused to resort to the traditional "pump 'em up" routine. A student of Tao Sports, Cindy chose to remain calm and focus her athletes, instead, on their inner divine feelings related to confidence, courage and passion. She told them: "You know, you may or may not win. Just have confidence in knowing you can play well, like the NCAA champs you are. Play with integrity and demonstrate your greatness; you will be winners regardless of the outcome." With this peaceful message and inner knowing that they could play with this kind of confidence, they went on to beat their nemesis by a score of 6–5. They "owned" the second half. When the game concluded, little was said about the obvious win; most of the talk was centered on the victory within, the internal triumph.

They learned to have confidence by simply exhibiting their presence, playing with their hearts and bonding with their souls; this was a confidence that they could control.

According to Tao, confidence or inner power is simply the influence you have over all situations in life. It is a state of being, an inner spiritual consciousness about your integrity as an athlete or person and your ability to exhibit this deeper self when necessary. Unlike the more traditional approach where confidence is tied to your thinking you can control the results or outcomes, the Tao way helps you to gather inner strength by focusing on the process and the moment-to-moment unfolding of events.

In Chinese, the word for confidence is "Zhai." Translated, it means a secure and peaceful place of being present, here and now. It is developed through years of practice by exhibiting a confidence of being totally comfortable with yourself, regardless of what you have achieved. You can sense this magnetism in great performers. Michael Jordan, Wayne Gretzky, Joe Montana and the great Pelé all have Zhai; they hold the audience spellbound with the singular high-voltage presence.

Ceci St. Géme had Zhai when she won the U.S. women's 5,000-meter national championship. As a student of Tao, she described her confidence as a peaceful, calm state that enabled her effort to seem almost too easy. She simply showed up to race with confidence in her ability to run like a world-class athlete.

Zhai, or inner confidence, can be detected in an opponent through their eyes, the windows to the soul. In an attempt to encourage his team to exhibit presence and display confidence, coach Mike Krzyzewski of the Duke University men's basketball program told his athletes prior to a crucial playoff game on the road to the Final Four, "There will be a point in the game tomorrow where they'll look you in the eye and what they see will determine the outcome." The Duke Blue Devils had fire in their eyes and went on to beat UNLV, the number-one team in the nation at that time.

Try to shift your consciousness about confidence to a deeper, more dynamic plane and apply it to your sports and exercise program. For example, refuse to simply show up at a contest or the gym to win or to look terrific; show up on a deeper level and perform according to your ability and exhibit your presence in this way. Gone will be the anxiety and tension that usually arrive when you try to be confident in winning. Focusing on your ability level alone will help you to feel inner strength, courage and Zhai—real, meaningful confidence.

Once you "get it" in your physical regimes, search for ways in which you can apply this inner universal truth to areas in life where confidence is an issue. For example, when talking to an audience, rather than obsess about your performance, get in touch with your essence, your purpose and your heart and simply deliver the message from an inner, more spiritual focus. You can't control how they feel about you or whether they like what you say, but you can control how you exhibit yourself as you perform with integrity. When applying for a job, for example, divert your attention away from how you look and focus, instead, on being yourself throughout the interview. Have confidence in the way you present yourself as a sincere, dedicated, reliable, dependable applicant.

If, after shifting your ideas about confidence in this way, you still feel a lack of confidence in sports or in life, seek the support and encouragement of a coach, a close friend and your family. Perhaps they can give you a realistic assessment about who you are and where you are at so that you can have a confident, realistic point of reference for your performance. Also, observe others with similar abilities and life situations such as yours. Their success and how they perform can give you the confidence that you, too, can perform with Zhai.

Use the following exercises to help you cultivate inner talent and to nurture and reinforce the power of exhibiting your presence. Remember, also, that you will want to precede your daily workout or sports activity with a ten-minute Tao Mind breathing and visualization session to help you relax and focus on how you wish to perform your exercise regimen:

## A. BREATH WATCHING

Again, in our relaxed Tao Mind state, with eyes closed:

- Inhale slowly through nostrils and watch with your eyes closed the "white cloud" fill the lungs completely.

- Suspend breath for a few seconds (three to five) and watch the clean air travel to all extremities of your body.

- Exhale and watch the "smoky de-oxygenated cloud" exit the nostrils as carbon dioxide. See it dissolve and disappear.

- Suspend breath for a few seconds (three to five) and imagine the emptiness of your lungs.

- Repeat this breath-watching process ten or more times and notice the calm relaxation take over.

### B. VISUALIZATION

Again, in your relaxed Tao Mind state, with eyes closed:

- *Visualize* a time when you felt extremely confident in your ability.

- *See* yourself about to partake in that sport, workout or performance.

- *Feel* confidence throughout your body being in control over how you now perform.

- *See* yourself as you exhibit a flawless presence, replicating the past experience.

- *Feel* your confidence level begin to soar as you float through the performance.

### C. AFFIRMATIONS

Remember that the following are samples of affirmations that reinforce the Tao lesson to be learned. On the blank lines provided, create some affirmations that are more personal and relevant to your journey. Experiment and have fun in the process and make good use of index cards, posting your affirmations in a variety of places. Also recite them to yourself during visualization and picture what the words actually say.

I am ready to exhibit and demonstrate my strength as an athlete (or anyone else).

Regardless of the score, I am so much more.

I possess all that I need to perform like a winner.

I feel secure and powerful right here, right now.

I am ready to show my power of being a winner.

I feel triumphant and I always play like a champion.

_____

_____

_____

## D. APPLICATION OF ANCIENT WISDOM

Use the following pragmatic shifts in attitude to help restructure your conceptual view of the world around you:

*Reach over your head with both arms wide open to feel the unlimited space above. Let the Qi power of the sky elevate your body from the crown of your head. Now circle your arms around the body to create a ring of light glowing with your presence. Open your eyes for panoramic vision, your heart to feel unlimited compassion, your gut to generate unlimited inner power. Feel the solid grounding of the earth below, and your inner golden fire aflame. From time to time, scoop in from all around, replenish the energy, the Qi into your inner furnace, your Dantien-belly.*

# The Wisdom of
# Non-Excessiveness

The *Tao Te Ching* advises how hoarding too much brings heavy loss. Excessiveness in any arena of life, according to this ancient Chinese wisdom, ushers in disorder and disaster leading to fatigue, illness, injury and burnout. It is the path of self-destruction. An inner practice demands non-excessive behavior patterns if meaning in life is to be found.

Sports and exercise bring vibrancy and wellness that makes for a healthier life, yet, excess in any way will strip you of the vitality accrued. The Taoist way to sidestep this potential disaster is *moderation,* the flowing dance between any two extremes. The Chinese calligraphic symbols for moderation interestingly point to the middle to prevent excess. Here is the wisdom of non-excessiveness.

As athletes and fitness enthusiasts, we are likely candidates to indulge in extremes of any sort; "more is better" seems to be the mantra of choice. A world-class marathoner was getting excellent results from his 110-miles-per-week training program. He qualified for the Olympic trials and hoped to make the U.S. team. He reasoned that if he got to this level by doing this much work, imagine how much better he'd be if he increased his mileage by forty to fifty miles each week. He followed this logic, self-destructed and never made it to the starting line. The problem here, as in other physical programs, is that the mind is always ready to tell the body to do more than it can handle.

The temptation to overextend with sports and fitness regimes is very enticing and attractive. However, all that you gain from being excessive is drastically offset by the accumulation of tightness, tension, stress, unbalance and fatigue, creating a debt that needs to be paid back with rest or you will eventually pay the price and collapse.

Many who train their bodies diligently are beginning to realize that not only are there spiritual and psychological advantages to moderation, but some important physiological benefits as well. For example, try to run, swim, bike or walk every other day, rather than seven days a week, and give your body a chance to recuperate and get even stronger; you can begin to use the "stress then rest" maxim for conditioning, alternating workout days with total days off in-between. If your team is constantly fatigued and overall performance is down, try reducing your workout time each day and notice the improvement in the results.

We know that truly good music is the result of the *space* between *notes*. The pause makes it what it is. Musical pauses are not a lack of action; they are an integral part of the action. So it is with your workout regime. Getting in good shape, regardless of your sport or activity, is the result of the *rest* (pause) or space between the workouts. Your cellular structure is fragile and requires periods of rest. You need to learn how to "fondle" your body into shape as opposed to excessively forcing or pushing it there.

Excessiveness, in a spiritual sense, is a cancer of the soul. It knocks you off balance, forces you to lose perspective on what's important and destroys your value structure at the cellular level. The perfect treatment for this illness is to fortify your spirit with moderation and inoculate your consciousness with a dose of "less is more." When this disease of excessiveness goes into remission, you begin to feel the physical, emotional and spiritual side effects. Motivation increases while excitement, joy, enthusiasm and satisfaction return. It brings you back, once again, to the pure spirit of play.

When you grasp the lesson of Tao, one of moderation, in sports and exercise, begin to see its application to other areas of your life. Too much work or too much play is far from the way of nature, the way things were meant to be. Focus on creating a life of balance with all that you do. Establish a list of your ten favorite things to do and attend to them each day. Such a list might include professional work, exercise, listening to music, playing with your kids, meditation, cooking a good meal, talking with a friend, sky watching and reading. Notice how you feel at the end of a day where you gave a moderate amount of time to each item. Balance in life is a deeply rewarding and delicious food for the soul. It makes you feel alive and aligned with your spirit, your higher, healthier, happier self.

With moderation and balance, you will notice how much easier life is when you have enough, as opposed to having more than enough. And how much more work and stress is required to achieve the latter? Leisure is important, yet in excess leads to restlessness and boredom. Work is crucial yet, in extreme, can cause havoc with other aspects of life. Social events are fun; if taken to extremes you'll become distracted and fatigued. Even with regard to diet, moderation with variation is the key.

Remember, a balanced, moderate life creates excitement and motivation coupled with unlimited possibilities for higher levels of functioning. The *Tao Te Ching* reminds us that the spiritually and emotionally evolved individual is one who avoids extremes, extravagance and excess. There is nothing better than moderation. There's an ancient Zen saying that seems appropriate here: moderation in all things, including moderation.

Use the following exercises to help you cultivate inner talent and to nurture and reinforce the wisdom of non-excessiveness. Remember, also, that you will want to precede your daily workout or sports activity with a ten-minute Tao Mind breathing and visualization session to help you relax and focus on how you wish to perform your exercise regimen:

## A. BREATH WATCHING

- Inhale slowly through nostrils and watch with your eyes closed the "white cloud" fill the lungs completely.

- Suspend breath for a few seconds (three to five) and watch the clean air travel to all extremities of your body.

- Exhale and watch the "smoky de-oxygenated cloud" exit the nostrils as carbon dioxide. See it dissolve and disappear.

- Suspend breath for a few seconds (three to five) and imagine the emptiness of your lungs.

- Repeat this breath-watching process ten or more times and notice the calm relaxation take over.

## B. VISUALIZATION

Again, in your relaxed Tao Mind state, with eyes closed:

- *See* a day in your life where you include most of your *Top Ten List.*

- *Taste* a bit of each item on your list.

- *Feel* fulfilled and satisfied going from one to the other with perfect balance.

- *See* yourself, at the end of the day, eating a delicious dinner, without overdoing it.

- *Feel* the elation of involving yourself in a variety of things, having it all with high energy.

## C. AFFIRMATIONS

Remember that the following are samples of affirmations that reinforce the Tao lesson to be learned. On the blank lines provided, create some affirmations that are more personal and relevant to your journey. Experiment and have fun in the process and make good use of index cards, posting your affirmations in a variety of places. Also recite them to yourself during visualization and picture what the words actually say.

Stress needs rest.

Less is, often, more.

Half empty is already half full!

I enjoy my repose with all the new spaces to be filled later.

_____

_____

_____

## D. APPLICATION OF ANCIENT WISDOM

Use the following pragmatic shifts in attitude to help restructure your conceptual view of the world around you:

> Two of the most treasured virtues of Tao wisdom are simplicity ("P'u") and modesty ("Jian"). Lao Tzu says in verses 57 and 67 of the TAO TE CHING, "I have no desires, and the people return to simplicity," and "Because I am modest, therefore I can be gregarious." Tai Ji practice helps us to work out in moderation, without falling into excessiveness. Enjoy the simple "at-ease-ness" of your practice, with a WINDFLOW quality to your motion. Before and after each physically demanding workout, put on some soothing and mellow music, move with it and feel the easy flowing Qi in and around your body.

# Lanterns Illuminating the Way

A sixty-year-old athlete had set a goal of running under three hours in the marathon. After thirteen unsuccessful attempts at his almost impossible task, a friend asked why he continued to attempt what seemed to be a futile ambition. Without a moment's hesitation, he stated that the attainment of the goal was not the objective; his kick was the elation he experienced in other parts of life from setting that goal: repeated months and years of joy, training at high levels, getting into great shape, eating well and feeling terrific. Nothing else in life could do that for him. The goal became simply a lantern that illuminated his way and, according to him, "kept me totally involved with health and wellness, a process relevant to my spiritual growth in all aspects of life."

Goals, from a Taoist perspective, are beacons that help to keep your soul on track and gain access into your deep passions. They are an integral component of an internal spirit quest, one that searches for and nurtures self-confidence and well-being. Goals help you to create a strong bond between what you dream and what you do.

In sports and exercise, once you begin to make this shift in consciousness, you open yourself up to opportunities to massage the spirit; you reduce unnecessary pressure and anxiety over trying to achieve the outcome or goal; you also cease to measure your self-worth based on the outcome and, therefore, nurture your self-esteem. The key is to set your goals in the spirit of passion, goals that are aligned with what you love, then proceed to enjoy thoroughly the process of following the direction they take you.

Three-time U.S. national vaulting champion Keri Lemon took a Tao Sport approach to her goal-setting process. She loved every aspect of her sport: the costumes, the music, the movement, the horse, the travel and social benefits. Her goal to win the world championship was more about a journey of inner fitness than about the gold medal. When she set the objective she knew that the lofty goal would enable her to continue her passion at an even higher level for a period of one year. Living the lifestyle of a champion, she went to Germany, placed second in the world, and immediately began to search for ways to repeat the process. By focusing on her process in this way, she not only had a great year, she was able to perform at a level no other American had ever come close to in a sport dominated by the Europeans.

When you think about it, many of your goals in life, even if achieved, were rarely as important as the experience itself on the path to that goal. Potters talk about how the treasure is not in the pottery, but in the experience of making it. The metaphor of a dancer is also a good example of this. When the dance is choreographed, the process is just beginning; then the dancer experiences the joy and relives this creative experience, fresh and new, over and over again. In both of these examples, the opportunity for self-renewal and growth is abundant as you enter into the meditative state of solitude and in-the-moment flow, free of the tension created by pushing toward an outcome.

When you begin to embrace this "new" ancient way in sports and exercise, notice how much better you feel about the setting of goals, free of anxiety and stress. Take how you feel and begin to apply this attitude to other situations in life.

Let's say that you are interested in writing a book. Rather than be nervous about the publishing process or the goal of completion, let the goal itself be a way to help you stay connected to yourself in a therapeutically, meditative state where you can relax and shut out the chatter of the world as you write. Perhaps you want to attain a black belt in aikido; let the goal become the excuse to enjoy the dance, movement and training as you refine your skills at the dojo. Notice too, when reading a great book that when the pleasurable process is over, you are saddened and search for another to help you replicate this good feeling. The goals, in these cases, become the guiding lights to keep you in the pleasurable process of attending to your great spirit, what makes you feel most alive.

Goals, therefore are beacons, dreams or lanterns that keep you on track. Be cautious of using a goal simply as a notch in your belt or something to achieve. This will detach you from the essence of sport, fitness and life's other activities. Let your goals simply be the vehicle to place you on an internal quest, one of complete enjoyment in the moment. To see them otherwise is to miss the point completely. Pushing or forcing your way to a fabricated destination is counterproductive.

Use the following exercises to help you cultivate inner talent and to nurture and reinforce the Tao approach to goals. Remember, also, that you will want to precede your daily workout or sports activity with a ten-minute Tao Mind breathing and visualization session to help you relax and focus on how you wish to perform your exercise regimen:

## A. BREATH WATCHING

Again, in our relaxed Tao Mind state, with eyes closed:

- Inhale slowly through nostrils and watch with your eyes closed the "white cloud" fill the lungs completely.

- Suspend breath for a few seconds (three to five) and watch the clean air travel to all extremities of your body.

- Exhale and watch the "smoky de-oxygenated cloud" exit the nostrils as carbon dioxide. See it dissolve and disappear.

- Suspend breath for a few seconds (three to five) and imagine the emptiness of your lungs.

- Repeat this breath-watching process ten or more times and notice the calm relaxation take over.

## B. VISUALIZATION

Again, in your relaxed Tao Mind state, with eyes closed:

- *Set* a goal in sports, exercise or life that will be a guide for joy.

- *Imagine* all that's required to approach that goal; what's involved?

- *Feel* the joy, fun, excitement that are part of this journey.

- *See* yourself grow and expand physically, emotionally, spiritually.

- *Feel* exhilarated living this lifestyle—what fun.

- *Remind* yourself that goal attainment is not as important as the joy on the path.

- *Search* for another goal to replace the one that's completed, and go for it.

## C.  AFFIRMATIONS

Remember that the following are samples of affirmations that reinforce the Tao lesson to be learned. On the blank lines provided, create some affirmations that are more personal and relevant to your journey. Experiment and have fun in the process and make good use of index cards, posting your affirmations in a variety of places. Also recite them to yourself during visualization and picture what the words actually say.

My goals are lighting up my way from Here and Now on.

I feel my passion illuminating my power from inside out.

I love the experience of my brightness and joy on my way to reaching my goal.

_____

_____

_____

## D. APPLICATION OF ANCIENT WISDOM

Use the following pragmatic shifts in attitude to help restructure your conceptual view of the world around you:

*The space between your eyebrows is often referred to as the third eye; in Chinese it is called "Inn-tang," the Seal of the Inner Sanctum. When we are truly focused, this eye is a clear beacon showing the way, beaming ahead for us. Meditate on this special eye and feel its power. Place your index finger in front of this third eye and direct the finger from there straight ahead. As you do, project your wishes and see the image of your accomplishment revealed vividly. Repeat this exercise several times; then go ahead and be happy with the result of your game or workout.*

# What You See, You Get

I was never really good in sports. In my younger days, the neighborhood kids would laugh at me. At the age of thirty-eight, I took up cycling to get into shape and shed some pounds. Now I'm hooked on a sport for the first time ever. I've been working at it diligently for four years and I still don't do well in races. I'd love to be better but I guess I can't. I'm too slow and awkward; I can't help it. I've always been that way. Really, I don't see myself as a cyclist. I don't know why. Have I reached my potential?

In our estimation, Ben has not reached his full potential and has created imaginary limits that become "real" barriers because he "sees" them that way. Because he believes his images, he will unlikely do what needs to be done to bring about an improvement in his performance. This is the crux of his challenge. Change the image, and the results will come.

According to ancient wisdom, your personal power is manifested when you become conscious of your true nature and capabilities and act accordingly. The Tao teaches that to do otherwise causes inner friction and problems.

An important element to enhance your ability to explore the boundaries of your unlimited potential is the image you have of yourself. You carry around with you a mental blueprint, a picture or image of your self, based on past performances or the opinions of others. This is commonly referred to as self-esteem. Since your central nervous system does not distinguish between this image and what's real, how you see yourself is interpreted as real and determines how you'll act and perform ninety percent of the time. In other words, what you "see" is what you get. If you imagine yourself as unathletic, you would refuse to enter an arena that places physical demands upon you. Seeing yourself as awkward or as a klutz creates a negative image that stops you from trying to do anything physical. You will tend to avoid physical activity and never give yourself the chance to develop. The "picture" creates the reality.

Sports and exercise, once again, become a testing ground, enabling you to improve and expand your definition of self. The physical path provides a direct inner conduit for the creation of a positive self-image. With sports and exercise, you are being constantly challenged to face your fears, fatigue, ego, self-doubt and courage. When you dig down deep and rise to the occasion, you discover the real you. You collect the data that begins to redefine the image of who you really are at this moment, not what others may say about you. When you learn about your true self through your experiences in sports and exercise, you can create a realistic portrait and begin to blossom and unfold like the Tao, like a natural process. Your athletic and exercise performances will begin to reflect the more expansive image you now own.

Humans are animals, natural athletes from birth, and animals are also naturally graceful and athletic. Through consistent physical activity, you begin to reclaim your animal power and refuse to accept the negative labels imposed upon you by others. What you need to do is visualize yourself as a naturally graceful person emerging from those old superimposed negative images. See and feel yourself coming into your own, beaming and dancing joyously in the sunlight.

We (Jerry and Chungliang) know that how we feel and what we know about ourselves are the direct results of our experiences in sports, exercise and martial arts. We have been able to apply all that we have learned about ourselves from our athletic, martial arts and dance experiences to every aspect of life, be it publishing, teaching or fathering. With fortified self-images from these physical activities, we move forward with confidence, knowing who we are and nothing more.

When you begin to get in touch with the deep inner sense of self through your physical activity, believe in it and take the time to cultivate this inner power. Be vigilant and refuse to abandon your true nature. Own and exhibit your real power, who you really are; recognize and appreciate it. When confused or in doubt, remember this pertinent ancient Chinese story of the stonecutter:

> The stonecutter was unappreciative of who he was. Seeing a wealthy merchant, he desired to be such. When he became one, he realized that with all this power, he still had to bow before the king; of course, he now wished to be king. And so it was, until he noticed how much the sun could make him uncomfortable with its heat. How powerful the sun is, he thought, so he became the sun until the

cloud showed its power by covering up the sun. He then became the powerful cloud until, one day, the mighty wind pushed him around. He then became the wind, which could do all except blow the powerful stone. He became the stone, more powerful than anything on earth. As he stood proudly in the wind, he asked what could be more powerful than a stone? As he looked down, he saw a stonecutter, pounding him with a chisel.

Believe in yourself. Sports and exercise will keep you in touch with your true spirit. Like the Tao, notice what this is and behave accordingly.

Use the following exercises to help you cultivate a strong self-image. Remember, also, that you will want to precede your daily workout or sports activity with a ten-minute Tao Mind breathing and visualization session to help you relax and focus on how you wish to perform your exercise regimen:

## A. BREATH WATCHING

Again, in our relaxed Tao Mind state, with eyes closed:

- Inhale slowly through nostrils and watch with your eyes closed the "white cloud" fill the lungs completely.

- Suspend breath for a few seconds (three to five) and watch the clean air travel to all extremities of your body.

- Exhale and watch the "smoky de-oxygenated cloud" exit the nostrils as carbon dioxide. See it dissolve and disappear.

- Suspend breath for a few seconds (three to five) and imagine the emptiness of your lungs.

- Repeat this breath-watching process ten or more times and notice the calm relaxation take over.

## B. VISUALIZATION

Again, in your relaxed Tao Mind state, with eyes closed:

- *Think* of a time when you really felt good about yourself and a performance.

- *Feel* the deep sense of personal power you get from this experience.

- *Imagine* yourself like this now.

- *Feel* the peace, comfort and satisfaction of being spiritually and physically fit.

- *Receive* recognition from others, supporting you at what you do.

- *See* yourself being surrounded by people who are warm and kind to you.

- *Feel* the love they offer and accept it in appreciation.

- *Tell* yourself that it's all good. Life is just fine.

## C. AFFIRMATIONS

Remember that the following are samples of affirmations that reinforce the Tao lesson to be learned. On the blank lines provided, create some affirmations that are more personal and relevant to your journey. Experiment and have fun in the process and make good use of index cards, posting your affirmations in a variety of places. Also recite them to yourself during visualization and picture what the words actually say.

I am authentic, unique and special. I like who I am.

Every day, in every way, I get better and better.

I am a natural athlete with surprising potentials.

I am delighted with what I envision, what I can do, and who I can be.

Sports and fitness activities are terrific opportunities to help me broaden and strengthen my self-image.

_____

_____

_____

## D. APPLICATION OF ANCIENT WISDOM

Use the following pragmatic shifts in attitude to help restructure your conceptual view of the world around you:

*Follow the same Tai Ji exercise in the previous goal-setting practice. First project your wishes ahead with focused vision into the bull's-eye screen. Now, pantomime the action of an accomplished Zen archer. Take the arrow out of the quiver, fit it properly on the string of the bow and point it to the bull's-eye. Enjoy what you see—the perfect image of yourself accomplishing your task. As you pull back the arrow, close your eyes and bring your focus back into your body and concentrate deep inside, from your brain, into your heart and down to your gut, your Dantien center. Be the image you see in your mind's eye, fully alive. Stretch the bow to its fullest, then release with a thunderous shout of confidence. You are IT!*

# Practice, Practice, Practice

According to the *Tao Te Ching*, those who achieve mastery are limitless. Mastery, a high level of proficient, competent, versatile wizardry, is available to all who enter any arena of play, regardless of past experiences. Your inability to rise to this level in prior times is not reason to prevent you from enjoying high masterful levels of participation now. If you presently have an activity that you wish to master, it is attainable through the natural process of noticing your shortcomings and doing what it takes to go beyond them: It takes *practice, practice and more practice.*

The Chinese Book of Change and Transformation, the *I Ching*, reminds you of how attention to detail, through practice, will allow you to accomplish anything. In sports and exercise, this means learning the fundamentals, the basics that help you to build a strong foundation to create your dream. The journey of mastery may be a thousand miles but it does require one small step at a time. Your success on this journey is measured by the quality of those steps, and your attention to the practice. Whatever your arena of choice in sports, fitness and life, practice consistently every day, and proficiency is yours. When you want to excel at anything, do not look for a quick fix; there are no immediate results.

The Chinese symbol for practice shows a young bird flapping its wings constantly until it learns to fly. When you wish to learn how to do your "flying" in sports and exercise, remember the metaphor of the bird. You must constantly repeat your practicing of a certain skill until your spirit takes flight, soaring with joy and enormous magnitude. And, no matter how good you get at your game, there's always the need for repetition with variation if you want to keep flying. A visible world-class athlete who seems to have no trouble flying and soaring is Michael "Air" Jordan. He keeps aloft his competitors because he insists on practicing continuously. Jordan has been known to show up early on game day and, in the absence of his teammates, work on his three-point shot, over and over until he nears perfection. If an athlete as great as Jordan understands the need to practice repeatedly, perhaps we all should consider its value in our physical endeavors. John Wooden, coach of the powerful UCLA Bruins basketball dynasty, says that the road to mastery is through the eight laws of learning: explanation, demonstration, imitation, repetition, repetition, repetition, repetition and repetition.

The physical act of repeated practice can be considered an excellent sacred mentor, creating opportunities for you to learn how to become calm and quiet as you focus on the process of repetitive motion. Practice becomes an in-the-moment, methodical, satisfying experience on the path of mastery. With practice you begin to notice steady, subtle, continual progress that is quite satisfying. Gains are inevitable with daily attention to learning any skill or technique. But it does take time and diligent work because there will be the plateaus along the way, periods of relative stability where there is little or no apparent progress or benefit. See this absence of progress as another important, necessary aspect to the upward learning curve. The plateau can be used as a natural pause, an important time of reflection, reevaluation, revelation and, perhaps, rest or hibernation, part of the periodic cycle where you level out before you spurt ahead. It is a sacred time, offering you the chance to work with your feelings of frustration and annoyance.

To help yourself with this period of stagnation, don't fight it or push it aside; see it for what it is, an essential step for anyone who chooses to be on the road to excellence. Be kind to yourself, like a good self-coach, and remember that breakthroughs are waiting in the wings. Here is your opportunity to experience how a calm and adaptable demeanor along with good-natured persistence will help you through this trying period to mastery and good fortune. Learn that becoming a good cyclist or becoming good at anything is the result of "time in the saddle," hours of practice even when you begin to level out and seem to be "spinning your wheels," getting nowhere. The master dancer, after a brilliant evening performance, goes right back to the bar at the studio first thing in the morning.

Trust that by practicing each day, especially during plateaus, you will store all that experience and *when called into action*, the body will *always* deliver the goods.

The same principles that apply to your physical life are relevant to all arenas of life as well. Once you understand the importance of practice and the function of plateaus on the journey of mastery in sports and exercise, it will make it easier to apply this understanding when you begin to learn how to type, write, paint, publish, speak, plant, build, sing or dance. Notice how patient and accepting you become of your slow, deliberate progress toward satisfaction and competency with your performance.

Now, before your attempt to practice anything, in a standing position, imagine yourself as a big bird: Feel yourself getting ready to take off (in any arena of life) with your winged potential. Breathe deeply, expand your chest to widen your shoulders and spread your arms for the uplifting sensation in your whole being. Imagine the moment when your spirit takes flight as you soar with joy.

Use the following exercises to help you cultivate inner talent and to nurture and reinforce the importance of practice. Remember, also, that you will want to precede your daily workout or sports activity with a ten-minute Tao Mind breathing and visualization session to help you relax and focus on how you wish to perform your exercise regimen:

## A. BREATH WATCHING

Again, in our relaxed Tao Mind state, with eyes closed:

- Inhale slowly through nostrils and watch with your eyes closed the "white cloud" fill the lungs completely.

- Suspend breath for a few seconds (three to five) and watch the clean air travel to all extremities of your body.

- Exhale and watch the "smoky de-oxygenated cloud" exit the nostrils as carbon dioxide. See it dissolve and disappear.

- Suspend breath for a few seconds (three to five) and imagine the emptiness of your lungs.

- Repeat this breath-watching process ten or more times and notice the calm relaxation take over.

## B. VISUALIZATION

Again, in your relaxed Tao Mind state, with eyes closed:

- *See* yourself during some practice session.

- *Imagine* repeating a certain routine over and over until it feels monotonous.

- *Shift* your consciousness and discover the joy and worth of repetitious movement.

- *Feel* yourself enjoying the plateau, a place to reflect your past and future potential.

- *Tell* yourself that breakthroughs are waiting to happen.

- *Feel* good about your new Tao approach to practice.

## C. AFFIRMATIONS

Remember that the following are samples of affirmations that reinforce the Tao lesson to be learned. On the blank lines provided, create some affirmations that are more personal and relevant to your journey. Experiment and have fun in the process and make good use of index cards, posting your affirmations in a variety of places. Also recite them to yourself during visualization and picture what the words actually say.

All things come my way when I practice every day.

I enjoy the way to mastery more than mastery itself.

Practice is a joy, my eternal delight.

_____

_____

_____

## D. APPLICATION OF ANCIENT WISDOM

Use the following pragmatic shifts in attitude to help restructure your conceptual view of the world around you:

*Tao helps us to renew each practice afresh and see each workout as a rediscovery of its many pleasures. With Tao, you can easily transcend the drudgery of repetitious routines. Use this easy Tai Ji self-spoofing exercise called "Kai-Hsing" (open your heart-*

*mind) to wake up to the here and now. Cross your arms in front of your chest, spread them open and glibly say to yourself: "Another LOUSY sunset in paradise!" Then, in your mind's eye, marvel at the breathtaking beauty of this repetitious miracle. Repeat this exercise several times. Practice, practice and practice your true awareness of the excitement of here and now, here and now, here and now, again and again!*

K A I

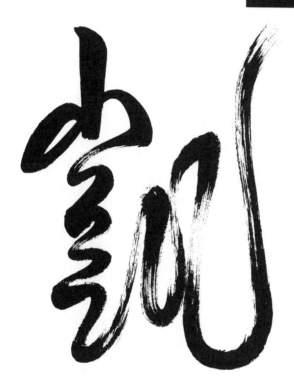

**Joy of triumphant spirit**
**Spinning on the mountain top**

*I*n traditional athletic and exercise programs, the field, court, track, health spa and training center are viewed as battlefields against an opponent, a score, a clock, a machine or yourself. The new Tao of Inner Fitness approach to sports and exercise views these venues as arenas for the battles *within*, opportunities to help you go inside, dig deep and learn about internal concerns such as fear, fatigue, failure, patience, persistence, perseverance, courage, commitment, confidence, self-doubt and ego. In this way, the physical becomes a sacred path of self-discovery and a meditative time to be with yourself. Here, in this stage of the journey, you'll learn through Chinese paradox, how loss is gain, and you begin to truly grasp the notion of failure as success. You will be given the chance to understand the real meaning of winning as you detach from outcomes and results. When you go inside and confront your self-doubts, you'll learn how vulnerabilities and shortcomings can be used to your advantage in a world of healthy competition. For those of us involved with team activities, interdependence, oneness, cooperation, devotion and loyalty are spiritual virtues that will guide you toward synergistic play. Your inner battles will take on new meaning as you become more familiar with Tao as the Watercourse Way, where you learn to yield, flow and blend with external forces through the act of nonresistance. Finally, you will discover the true benefit of being humble in your endeavors as you learn how to sidestep the tendency to be smitten with your progress.

The overall guiding message at this point is the thought that external victory of any kind, whether it's winning a game, securing

169

a contract, passing an exam, getting a job, being the champion in your field, is simply a reflection of inner triumph. When the memories of winning trophies and medals have faded, the victories over the inner demons will remain alive; the awards are the by-products of having had the courage to fail and the patience and perseverance to handle a misguided ego and your struggle with self-doubt.

The formula is simple: With inner success, there is less need for external victory. With less need for external victory, you experience less tension, anxiety and stress. With less anxiety, tension and stress, you naturally achieve your best external results. Success in this life, therefore, is the luminous reflection of all the inner victories you experience through sports and physical activity; it is a coming to terms with your innermost self and how that impacts your entire world as you feel it deep within your soul.

Throughout this stage, you will begin to view the physical path in an even broader spiritual way in which the real challenge is within, the opponent is yourself, and the reward is very personal and private. All results and outcomes in your world are now seen as the by-products of having met the challenge.

Let's say that your are confronted with the notion of failure or setback during a game or workout. Ask yourself: "What is the situation demanding of me? What do I need to rely on to meet this challenge? What am I made of that will enable me to take this on? How can I turn this situation around so that I can benefit from it?" Answering these questions helps you to better meet the real challenge inside. The chapters in this stage will help you to rise to the occasion and become victorious with the battles within. To set the tone, consider the following story about a soccer athlete who was playing his first game and was frightened over the prospect of defeat:

On the morning of his first game, Danny went to his coach and told him his concern about the opposition scoring too many goals with him in the nets. His coach told Dan how the best goalies in the world get scored upon and that puts him in good company. He further reassured Dan that whether they score or not, he can still *play* like a champion, diving for balls, jumping high to deflect shots, and staying alert throughout the game. Finally, he told him to have fun in the execution of this plan and if he didn't have fun, he wouldn't play another game with this team. With the pressure off, Dan allowed only one goal, but the opposition won the game 1–0. Even in loss, everyone vigorously applauded Dan's heroics, courageousness and enthusiasm. He was a winner even though the score didn't reflect it. Danny felt proud of his "winning" performance. Playing like a winner, regardless of the outcome, is a sure path to winning for a lifetime. Dan experienced a victory that most people would never read about in the sports pages.

# With No Need to Win,
# Victory Is Yours

From a Taoist perspective, a winner is one who, paradoxically, lets go of the need to win and, in the process, becomes victorious. Ancient wisdom encourages you to focus on the dance and be the best dancer you can be at that particular moment. The true reward of every sports or exercise program is experienced *now*, in the moment-to-moment excellence that you choose to exhibit. According to the Tao, attachments to outcomes detract and diminish your strength and personal power. When an athlete has a need to win, anxiety and tension flourish. The pressure to control the outcome causes physiological restrictions as muscles become more tight and less fluid.

Such had been the case with speed skater Dan Jansen, world record holder in the 500 meters. In seven consecutive Olympic races, he had failed to medal even though he was the overwhelming favorite to win. But there was one last chance for victory before he would decide to retire from competition. Unlike in the previous seven races where he had accepted the pressure and needed to win, he decided to simply show up for the 1,000-meter race and skate in

a relaxed state and let go of the need to control the outcome. To inoculate himself against the "need to win" virus, he focused on the
dance of the race, racing like a world champion, not on the
prospect of winning the gold. By following this Tao-like inner-
directed tack he was able to neutralize his anxiety and skate to levels unexpected. The shift in consciousness from "I must win" to "I
may or may not win, but I'll skate like a world-class athlete" enabled Jansen to win the gold in record time and end the long saga
of futility. He was victorious during the journey and the by-
product, as in all arenas of life, was triumph on the scoreboard. His
performance could actually be considered a form of meditation in
which he could stay calm, focus on the moment and make things
happen.

Someone once asked, "If winning isn't important, why keep
score?" Well, it is important and a great deal of fun. Yet, winning
should not be an end in itself, although many would disagree. For
some, the thought of victory is more important than life itself and
many literally are willing to kill themselves to get to the winner's
circle. Witness the wide use of anabolic steroids, a deadly drug, by
top athletes who would sell their souls for a win. We are taught
from an early age to focus externally, and if we win, somehow we
will be happy and our life will be great. Winning, according to
some people, may even make you a better human being. All of this
reasoning, of course, is sheer nonsense.

Such thought processes are widespread not only in sports, but
are the trend in many arenas of modern life. Much of our social
structure is built around the antiquated notion that there's no room
for second place. This attitude is substantiated by many athletes
competing in the Olympic games. According to many narrow, destructive minds, "You don't win silver, you lose gold." This heart-

less emphasis on winning (being named first overall or first in age division, or gaining some external reward) can damage your spirit and rob your soul; it can be physically and psychologically harmful as well. It adds unnecessary layers of tension, anxiety and stress, which contribute to unfavorable outcomes and the ability to do your best. When obsessed with winning, your body is unable to move with the fluidity or flow that's so necessary for winning performances. With a mind fixed tightly on outcomes, the body becomes extremely rigid. With a free-flowing mind, the body flows freely. Letting go of the rigid need to win is a sure way to reduce the anxiety, thus increasing the chances of victory.

To help divert your attention away from results and outcomes during any arena of performance, consider the following story. A professional athlete in the National Basketball Association was concerned about a crucial upcoming game and wanted to relieve himself of the tension and anxiety created over trying to control the outcome. He kept getting worrisome, negative thoughts, practically seeing himself self-destruct during the contest. We suggested that he make a list of the five ways he could play like a champion, to be his best in each moment of the game. Among those items on the list was to hustle, to guard his opponent tightly with arms raised high, to look for the open shot and take it, to watch the game, not the coach or crowd, and to breathe deeply and concentrate on the rotation of the ball prior to releasing a foul shot. We asked that he consider himself a successful athlete if he played according to this plan and had fun in the execution of each item. His focus was so narrowed that he never once thought about the results. He was a huge success, and played an excellent game, even though his team fell short of the win. The point is, you too can divert your concerns about outcomes to concerns about the process. As a result, you will perform at higher levels as well. Choose five ways in which you can perform your best with a certain task. For example, perform your task with proper form. Make it a point to breath properly. Use visualization prior to the execution of a particular skill. Perform in a relaxed fashion. Perhaps you can communicate clearly to those around you. Let the outcomes be the by-products of how you perform these five items moment to moment. Prepare properly by focusing on doing your best; you may not win but you will never lose.

In life, "winning" might be landing a job, receiving a contract, reaching a quota, passing an exam, entering a graduate program, gaining approval. Go about these tasks with your heart rather than your head. Again seize the opportunity to grow internally and let go of any dire need to win. Take it to another level spiritually by refusing to measure your self-worth by the outcome. Know that you are much more complex and important than a simple game, event or routine. Rather than trying to "win," simply demonstrate your ability to perform up to your capability—nothing more, nothing less. It's healthy to maintain your desire for triumph, but realize that you don't really "need" it; victory is an illusion of happiness that rarely fulfills its promise. With this inner awakening, you will immediately reduce your anxiety and, paradoxically, increase the chances of victory in the process. Focus, instead, upon performing the best you can; redefine "winning" as the ability to exhibit your skills and talents learned during your lifetime. Think about this: When one eye is on winning or outcomes, there's only one left to focus on the moment. Tell yourself this truth: Your greatest triumphs are always the by-products of your ability to demonstrate the level you have attained in anything you do. Focus on the moment, the experience itself, rather than how successfully you arrive.

Know, too, that external results are ephemeral; internal victory lasts forever.

Use the following exercises to help you cultivate inner talent and to nurture and reinforce the concept of true victory. Remember, also, that you will want to precede your daily workout or sports activity with a ten-minute Tao Mind breathing and visualization session to help you relax and focus on how you wish to perform your exercise regimen:

## A.  BREATH WATCHING

Again, in our relaxed Tao Mind state, with eyes closed:

- Inhale slowly through nostrils and watch with your eyes closed the "white cloud" fill the lungs completely.

- Suspend breath for a few seconds (three to five) and watch the clean air travel to all extremities of your body.

- Exhale and watch the "smoky de-oxygenated cloud" exit the nostrils as carbon dioxide. See it dissolve and disappear.

- Suspend breath for a few seconds (three to five) and imagine the emptiness of your lungs.

- Repeat this breath-watching process ten or more times and notice the calm relaxation take over.

## B. VISUALIZATION

Again, in your relaxed Tao Mind state, with eyes closed:

- *Imagine* yourself as you perform your physical activity up to your capability.

- *Feel* the confidence that's yours as you perform extremely well.

- *Feel* the thrill that comes from demonstrating your personal high-level performance.

- *Experience* the fun as you execute the plan as envisioned.

- *Feel* pride from your efforts.

- *See* yourself as a winner in all of life.

## C. AFFIRMATIONS

Remember that the following are samples of affirmations that reinforce the Tao lesson to be learned. On the blank lines provided, create some affirmations that are more personal and relevant to your journey. Experiment and have fun in the process and make good use of index cards, posting your affirmations in a variety of places. Also recite them to yourself during visualization and picture what the words actually say.

Win or lose, I play, run, ski, study, prepare like a champion.

I am victorious because I feel this way.

Winning is only the outcome: Doing what I love to do is the real thing!

Winning in sport and life is the joy in the execution of a well-defined plan.

_____

_____

_____

## D.  APPLICATION OF ANCIENT WISDOM

Use the following pragmatic shifts in attitude to help restructure your conceptual view of the world around you:

> *"By not presuming to be ahead of others, one can fulfill his potential best at last" (TAO TE CHING, verse 67). In Tai Ji practice, stepping back to create more open perspective while sinking low to experience higher space are norms. Everything is relative. To fully experience accomplishment in your workout, the only competitor is the true self you can become. Find the winner within by the example of the gesture of the infant Buddha. Stand up. Raise your right arm up, pointing to the sky; your left arm and finger pointing to earth. Stretch yourself and pronounce for all to hear: "Worlds above! And Worlds below! The Chief of all the worlds am I!"*

# Loss Is Gain

While the highly ranked University of Kentucky men's basketball team (second in the nation) seemed shaken by an unexpected home-court loss to South Carolina, their coach, Rick Pitino, wasn't. He sifted through the slaughter, made the necessary adjustment and focused his team on the setback as a lesson in attitude. He embraced the loss as a teacher, instructing them about their shortcomings and the healthy changes they needed to make. From that point on, they breezed through the 1997 NCAA tournament, making it to the finals for the second consecutive year only to lose a close match to the University of Arizona.

The *Tao Te Ching* mentions how we profit through loss. Times of advancement are always preceded by times of chaos. Success comes to all who can see their way out of the storm. Lao Tzu taught that we must regard failure, setbacks and mistakes as lessons from which to learn. Three-time Olympic gold medalist Jackie Joyner-Kersee followed this advice. She claims that losing, for her, was extremely valuable; understanding her setbacks allowed her to go on and win.

After a heartbreaking defeat in a recent NCAA basketball road to the Final Four tournament, a wise coach stated that although his team's setback was a loss in the physical world, it was a triumph in the spiritual realm. According to him, they learned from the loss and became a more solid, unified team.

When you see loss with an internal shift in consciousness, it opens your heart to a more compassionate, understanding approach to loss or failure; we've been told from birth that failure is an abomination, to be avoided at all cost. Traditionally, athletes and exercise enthusiasts become devastated in the wake of "undesirable" results. When you adopt a more natural, softer Tao approach to adversity, you cease to abuse yourself emotionally and create an inner environment where self-forgiveness can open the door for exploration into the sea of your vast potential. Accepting failure as a necessary aspect to success enables you to try and try again, learning from each setback until you master the task. Using a metaphor from nature, remember that because of the adverse conditions in a forest, a tree is forced to push its way upward to great heights. Times of adversity, in all of life, are periods of great blossoming as a person and as an athlete.

Sports and exercise give us plenty of opportunity to practice the Tao and become internally at peace with failure and loss. Everyone experiences setbacks; they cannot be avoided. It is said there are two kinds of performers in the world: Those who fail and those who will. Acceptance of this fact will help you to be more accepting of your shortcomings, not only in sports, but in all of life. Great athletes and performers become winners because they seem to have a very high tolerance for failure. They win even in defeat and see these moments of crisis through the eyes of a Taoist. In

Chinese, the word for crisis means two things simultaneously: danger and opportunity. Your failures are timely opportunities for you to grow internally through self-acceptance and learn what needs to be learned, and then, with your new knowledge, improve and forge ahead. You did this as a child when you mastered walking, a physical skill exponentially more complex than any skill you're trying to learn now. You did so by repeatedly correcting errors even though you experienced tremendous pain in the process. Failure was your teacher, and you learned well. All physical skills such as walking are perfected through adversity and failure.

Now, let's say that you've recently experienced a major setback in your physical program. After you've handled your disappointment and realized that you're like every other great athlete in this way, identify what you have learned in defeat and begin to see how this will help you to progress to a higher level in the future. Your positive reaction to what was once a hostile situation is indicative of how spiritually fit you are becoming.

It may also help you to notice how it is absolutely impossible for anyone to be thoroughly successful, competent and achieving in school, business or other performance arenas. To think otherwise is extremely irrational and the cause of much inner turmoil. When you find yourself feeling a void after a setback in life, tell yourself that ups and downs are nature's way; you win some, you lose some. It may be healthy to take ourselves less seriously. Refuse to fight with yourself when this teacher pays an unexpected visit. Open up to learning from this well-intentioned "coach."

Consider being like the Zen Warrior: Expect nothing but be ready for anything. If you have high expectations with regard to outcomes, you are setting yourself up for setbacks. You can try to establish strong visions of preference and then do everything within your ability and power to bring those preferences to fruition. This way, loss will not be so devastating.

Use the following exercises to help you cultivate an acceptance of failure, as a teacher in all of life. Remember, also, that you will want to precede your daily workout or sports activity with a ten-minute Tao Mind breathing and visualization session to help you relax and focus on how you wish to perform your exercise regimen:

### A. BREATH WATCHING

Again, in our relaxed Tao Mind state, with eyes closed:

- Inhale slowly through nostrils and watch with your eyes closed the "white cloud" fill the lungs completely.

- Suspend breath for a few seconds (three to five) and watch the clean air travel to all extremities of your body.

- Exhale and watch the "smoky de-oxygenated cloud" exit the nostrils as carbon dioxide. See it dissolve and disappear.

- Suspend breath for a few seconds (three to five) and imagine the emptiness of your lungs.

- Repeat this breath-watching process ten or more times and notice the calm relaxation take over.

## B. VISUALIZATION

Again, in your relaxed Tao Mind state, with eyes closed:

- *Recall* a recent setback, mistake or failure in your life.

- *Replay* it in your mind's eye, this time correcting the situation.

- *See* how much better you perform from learning the lesson.

- *Feel* the exhilaration from doing it right, according to plan.

## C. AFFIRMATIONS

Remember that the following are samples of affirmations that reinforce the Tao lesson to be learned. On the blank lines provided, create some affirmations that are more personal and relevant to your journey. Experiment and have fun in the process and make good use of index cards, posting your affirmations in a variety of places. Also recite them to yourself during visualization and picture what the words actually say.

My setbacks teach me to move forward.

Adversity gives me inner strength. I feel stronger.

Not winning is not the end. I take it all in and learn.

Defeat is the perfect mentor of all my future successes.

_____

_____

_____

## D. APPLICATION OF ANCIENT WISDOM

Use the following pragmatic shifts in attitude to help restructure your conceptual view of the world around you:

*Tao philosophy wisely states: "Every loss is a gain." It is best experienced by the Tai Ji move of emptying. First, gesture scooping with both hands from both sides of the body, to gather energy to fill your Dantien full of Qi. Take a deep inhaling breath to fortify this fullness of being. Feel the limit of oversaturation. Then exhale and release your fullness with swinging open arms. Experience how this reopened emptiness is regaining even more fresh fullness with new delight.*

# The Art of
# Seeking Together

The *I Ching* reminds us how working together helps us to achieve significant things. Synergistic interaction, according to Tao, provides an abundance of energy for continued expansion and growth. In sports and exercise programs, your opponents are valuable gifts, great teachers who can push you to physical, emotional and spiritual places you might not attain without them. By shifting your consciousness, competitors can become partners in a synergistic culture where everyone becomes a winner as you assist each other on the path of optimal performance. Your competitors are like spiritual advisors, helping you dig down deep and understand yourself more fully as they help bring out your best. Interestingly enough, when you trace the derivation of the word *compete,* you discover that it means "seek together." We truly have been derailed from this aspect of play.

In Chinese, the symbol for competitors shows many individuals helping each other share the same task. All your competitors are here to help you seek together to do your individual best, to push you to greater heights as you do the same for them. Invite and welcome this partnership.

Here is a fitting example of "seeking together." In the middle of a steep climb during a race a female pro cyclist felt that she was doing the best she could. At that moment, two opponents came from behind and began to pass her. Her first reaction was to quit; they were too strong and she'd get dropped. Then she remembered the concept of partnership and asked herself, "What can I do *now*? How can I let them help me?" She decided to not let them take off but chose, instead, to allow these athletes to "pull" her up the hill for only one minute. By staying with it for even a short period, she discovered reservoirs of strength and energy she had not known she had and regained her lead before the crest of the hill; she went on to win the race. Without them, she would never have dug so deep. Like all competitors, her opponents gave her an opportunity to go inside and see what she had left; they were gifts in disguise, even though, ostensibly, they were all focused on their own performance.

I (Jerry) can remember competing in a national championship fifteen-kilometer cross-country race in Houston. Most of the athletes were thinking of the ways they could defeat their closest rivals. They talked about the "killer instinct" and how important it was to compete well. I went up to the pre-race favorite and shocked him by saying, "I hope you have a great race." Confused and somewhat baffled by the words, he inquired as to why I felt that way. I told him, "The better you do, the better I will, too." He won the race and I claimed third, running my fastest time for the distance and pushing him to his greatest win in the process. We were seekers together on a path of self-discovery. Each of us was discovering something about who we were and how to take things up a notch.

It was a partnership of the heart, one where we offered each other, with intense competitive spirit, lessons about being a champion, a courageous opponent.

Focusing on diminishing others in order to make yourself appear larger than you are is a counterproductive, heartless path that takes away from, rather than contributes to, who you are and how you perform. This is easily illustrated by the following exercise: Draw a one-inch line on a piece of blank paper. Now, what can you do to make it look smaller or less than it is? Many of us will erase some of it; others will fold the paper in half; some will move the paper into the distance. These techniques do the job, yet cause you to focus lots of energy on that line. Instead, draw a five-inch line next to it and notice how the first line naturally looks smaller with respect to the new line. This is no different in competitive situations in sports and in life. When you enter the arena of competition, rather than focus on how to reduce the "enemy," concentrate on what you can do to make yourself better and how you can rise above to a higher dynamic plane. You can do this by using more effective tactics, improving your skills, trying better equipment, practicing more effectively and regarding your opponent as someone to treasure. All of these will "lengthen your line" of self-growth and improvement.

Furthermore, when you begin to feel anxious or tense during life's competitive situations, know that, like all of sports, it is a contest. In Latin, the word for "to contest" means to "testify with." Let your competitors be special witnesses to what you do; you must take a pledge to do your best. By entering such contests, you give your word to "put it on the line" and then allow your opponent to testify whether or not you have fulfilled your agreement. Being a good competitor yourself, you should sincerely thank the opposition for keeping you honest. And, in turn, you must offer to them the opportunity to take the same pledge and become their judge, to keep them honest. You are both there to teach each other this dance. It is a chance to exhibit your ability to display the sacred virtues of trust, reliability, dependability, integrity and interdependence.

Use the following exercises to help you cultivate inner talent and to nurture and reinforce the concept of opponent as partner. Remember, also, that you will want to precede your daily workout or sports activity with a ten-minute Tao Mind breathing and visualization session to help you relax and focus on how you wish to perform your exercise regimen:

## A. BREATH WATCHING

Again, in our relaxed Tao Mind state, with eyes closed:

- Inhale slowly through nostrils and watch with your eyes closed the "white cloud" fill the lungs completely.

- Suspend breath for a few seconds (three to five) and watch the clean air travel to all extremities of your body.

- Exhale and watch the "smoky de-oxygenated cloud" exit the nostrils as carbon dioxide. See it dissolve and disappear.

- Suspend breath for a few seconds (three to five) and imagine the emptiness of your lungs.

- Repeat this breath-watching process ten or more times and notice the calm relaxation take over.

## B. VISUALIZATION

Again, in your relaxed Tao Mind state, with eyes closed:

- *Imagine* anyone with whom you compete with in your life.

- *Feel* the connection you have as partners on this journey.

- *Tell* yourself, you are both here to teach each other lessons about life through sport.

- *Feel* relaxed and exhilarated as you challenge each other to greater heights.

- *Sense* the mutual respect and appreciation from having helped each other to greater heights.

- *Look* into each other's eyes with admiration.

## C. AFFIRMATIONS

Remember that the following are samples of affirmations that reinforce the Tao lesson to be learned. On the blank lines provided, create some affirmations that are more personal and relevant to your journey. Experiment and have fun in the process and make good use of index cards, posting your affirmations in a variety of places.

Also recite them to yourself during visualization and picture what the words actually say.

> I embrace all my opponents. They challenge me to perform better.
>
> My competitors are my mirrors. I see how much better I can be.
>
> Let's play together and achieve so much more.
>
> I'm here to help all of you to raise your level of performance.

---

---

---

## D. APPLICATION OF ANCIENT WISDOM

Use the following pragmatic shifts in attitude to help restructure your conceptual view of the world around you:

*Tai Ji practice may seem solitary, but it is never alone. We borrow forces from the sky, the earth, the environment and the vibration of others within our awareness. By tuning in to all around us, we learn to harness the Qi and make the best use of our workout, not as a chore, but as art and creative fun. Rhythm is the key. Experience yourself as a member of the full orchestra, co-creating beautiful music together. Or, as a member of a huge choir, be-*

coming all the voices. In front of the ocean, you are but one of the waves. Inside the forest, one of the trees. Stand up, be one of the multitude and share the collective power. Then move on to your sport or workout; be a thread interweaving with the tapestry of the surrounding rhythm.

# One Heart, One Goal

Ancient wisdom teaches how Heaven and Earth join spontaneously to create soft rain and gentle flowers. The Chinese calligraphic symbol for cooperation represents a oneness of vision sharing one heart and one reason. The *I Ching* reminds us about the importance of creating unity: The human spirit is nourished by a sense of connectedness.

So it is in your experience with teammates and training buddies in sports and fitness. With a mutual good sense for working together, the team and human spirit is enhanced and strengthened. You can begin to see how having a reliable training partner to meet you on cold mornings in the pool, or to "spot" you while pumping iron can be beneficial. Cyclists effectively use team members to draft for them, creating aerodynamic efficiency and, ultimately, better performance results. Unlike the previous chapter, "The Art of Seeking Together," which focused on competition, this chapter emphasizes how teammates and training partners can begin to perform at higher levels when they possess a unified purpose—cooperation and an attitude of interdependence.

Such unified purpose is best exemplified by the world champion Chicago Bulls professional basketball team. There are numerous stars on the squad, any one of whom could be selfish and dominate. Yet with single purpose of intent, under the leadership of coach Phil Jackson, they work selflessly together to connect spiritually with something bigger and better than themselves. Jackson, when he took over the Bulls, vowed to create an environment based on the principles of selflessness and compassion, virtues he had learned from his early Christian upbringing and the practice of Zen in his adult years. According to Phil, creating a successful team is essentially a spiritual act, one that requires all participants to forego self-indulgence for the greater good of the team. The Bulls have plugged into this power of oneness, and in the process of playing as a unit, they have set an all-time record for most victories in a single season, and have won five world championships on their way to being, arguably, the best team ever in the history of the NBA. Ancient wisdom tells us that the key to triumph is cooperation. The Taoist expert on strategy, Sun Tzu, believed that triumph is the result of unity of purpose and heart. The Bulls certainly exemplify the Tao in this way.

Unity of purpose and heart can be easily experienced through sports and exercise, which then opens the door to deeper spiritual growth. For example, notice how your workouts with a friend create the opportunity for both of you to connect in a stronger way. You tend to feel a bit closer, emotionally, to a friend when you run a few trails on a mountain together. When the two of you unite for the mutual purpose of discovering the unlimited boundaries of your potential, the physical exertion itself opens emotional, spiritual pathways that life, otherwise, may not permit you to enter. The bond grows deep and wide as you share a common purpose. On this physio-internal journey together, you become less self-absorbed as you show a willingness to give and receive on a higher level emotionally.

Teamwork and synergistic connectedness in the physical realm also help you to begin to understand the spiritual art of interdependence. You begin to realize that we are all connected to each other like the parts of a body; we are largely the sum total of all aspects of our life. The paper, taken from the tree, which grew from the soil, nurtured by the rain, was processed in the mill by a machine made from steel, mined by a person who reads the book created by the author who, and on and on and on. The key to fostering this strong connection is to keep from being self-centered by realizing your interdependence with others in all that you do. Also, know that you are capable of being so much more by opening up to the concept of interdependence.

Experiencing the countless spiritual benefits of one heart, one goal from your physical world should encourage you to look for ways to continue such synergistic activity in other arenas of life. The Tao encourages all of us to strive for togetherness to help us to go beyond our petty differences and to reunite our hearts in order to live in peace and harmony.

In the professional arena, notice how much greater your efforts can be when you connect with another and take your work to the next level. Our own successful cooperative writing collaboration has helped us to create and produce much more as a partnership, and with greater joy, than if we had tried to do it alone.

The Tao, talking about the cooperative efforts of Heaven and Earth, says that they are eternal and everlasting because they do not exist for themselves.

Use the following exercises to help you cultivate inner talent and to nurture and reinforce cooperation and unity of purpose. Remember, also, that you will want to precede your daily workout or sports activity with a ten-minute Tao Mind breathing and visualization session to help you relax and focus on how you wish to perform your exercise regimen:

## A. BREATH WATCHING

Again, in our relaxed Tao Mind state, with eyes closed:

- Inhale slowly through nostrils and watch with your eyes closed the "white cloud" fill the lungs completely.

- Suspend breath for a few seconds (three to five) and watch the clean air travel to all extremities of your body.

- Exhale and watch the "smoky de-oxygenated cloud" exit the nostrils as carbon dioxide. See it dissolve and disappear.

- Suspend breath for a few seconds (three to five) and imagine the emptiness of your lungs.

- Repeat this breath-watching process ten or more times and notice the calm relaxation take over.

## B. VISUALIZATION

Again, in your relaxed Tao Mind state, with eyes closed:

- *Imagine* yourself as an integral part of a team or group.

- *See* yourselves give support to each other, cooperating to bring out the best in each other.

- *Feel* the joy and camaraderie as you work synergistically from your hearts.

- *Hear* encouraging words from your partners, team members, colleagues.

- *Feel* yourself touch another in a positive, affirming way.

- *Give* praise to others in the group for their diligent efforts.

- *Notice* how others reciprocate your cooperative behavior.

- *See* all performances begin to soar.

## C. AFFIRMATIONS

Remember that the following are samples of affirmations that reinforce the Tao lesson to be learned. On the blank lines provided, create some affirmations that are more personal and relevant to your journey. Experiment and have fun in the process and make good use of index cards, posting your affirmations in a variety of places. Also recite them to yourself during visualization and picture what the words actually say.

Together, we are so much more.

I experience exultation when I cooperate with others.

I hear my single voice becoming all voices — a big resounding YES!

_____

_____

_____

## D. APPLICATION OF ANCIENT WISDOM

Use the following pragmatic shifts in attitude to help restructure your conceptual view of the world around you:

> Review the one-among-the-multitude exercise in the previous section on seeking together. There is only one cosmic hum. It is in the Chinese concept of heart-mind, nondivisional wholeness—Hsing. It is depicted as the stamen, the inner consciousness of every blossom in nature. The goal of improving our physical well-being is to enlighten our innermost emotional and spiritual well-being, sharing one heart of humanity.

# Resistance Creates
# Persistence

Anything that yields in life is more lasting than that which is rigid;
the nonresistant triumphs over the inflexible. These lessons from
the Tao point us to the path of least resistance, the Watercourse
Way. The Chinese character for yielding illustrates the way rivers
and streams form their paths according to the natural contours of
the land, suggesting that we go along and enjoy the flow.

In the Chinese movement art Tai Ji, one's motion is yielding
and nonresistant, a soft approach demonstrated by the Tui Shou
dance of pushing hands between two partners. Unlike its Western
counterpart of handshaking, a process of oversqueezing and cutting off intimacy, Tui Shou is an unforced blending together of
hands in circular fashion: When pushed, you pull; when pulled, you
push. Resistance of a force creates persistence of conflict and tension resulting in chaos. Resistance creates an energy drain while
yielding conserves it.

Unlike the earlier chapter "Effort Without Effort," in which
the objective is to help you see the benefits of applying less force,

this chapter on resistance is here to help you yield to any force or conflict that may stand in your way.

As you may know, all great athletes inevitably experience slumps; they cannot be avoided. However, if anyone tries to resist or force them away, they create extreme pressure and tension, intensifying the situation and extending its hold. You can see an athlete's frustration mount as he or she begins to push and force the shot, the swing, the stroke, the throw. To turn it around, you need to relax and yield. If you resist, it will persist. When an all-American lacrosse athlete was having difficulty finding the goal, she was advised to let the game come to her. She needed to notice the pace of the game and adjust to its flow; she would then be in better position to score. The very next game she let the game evolve at its own speed, blended with the flow and scored the winning goal with four minutes to play. She learned the lesson of noticing the flow and yielding to its power.

Sports and exercise can teach you valuable inner teachings about the power of yielding and not forcing. If you feel yourself resisting what is or forcing what's not, follow the Tao and be flexible; consider adapting to what comes your way, even if contrary to your wishes, and you will experience greater peace and calm. For example, let's say that you're an archer or a golfer. Notice nature by taking into consideration the wind factor while aiming at the target. To fight or resist nature's way is pointless, creates turmoil and is self-defeating. To get upset over what's happening is to fuel the fires of anger and frustration. If you are a mountain-bike athlete, you may consider trying to yield to the slope of the hill rather than trying to fight or conquer it. In the midst of a basketball game, you may be wiser to let things happen naturally; observe the flow and let the game come to you rather than trying hard to force every single aspect of play. Trying to "make it happen" creates tension and stress. Yielding to a force and exerting your presence will make you feel relaxed and put you at ease. When angry at an opponent, referee or situation that is beyond your control, know that you defeat yourself when you lose your temper, your "Tai Ji cool" as it were. Force always creates a counter force. Refuse to meet a force head on. There is no need to out-force an opponent when you can out-smart him or her.

With physical activity, you can learn the spiritual benefits of yielding when you become vulnerable to injury. Like anything else in life, if you resist, it will persist. When you get injured with sports or exercise, see an opportunity to expand spiritually as the injury gives you time to reflect upon your training or life. Perhaps something is not right; yield to it by accepting and learning from the situation. We suggest during this downtime that you go deep inside and reevaluate what you are doing and how you go about it. Maybe you are overtraining without taking the required rest periods. If you feel fatigued, rather than fight it or get uptight—yield. Acknowledge it is as a necessary step in the exploration of your unlimited potential, a natural response to exertion. By so doing, you'll relax and perform at higher levels.

So it is in all of life. Sometimes events and circumstances are contrary to our plans and desires, causing inner strife. Most of your conflict can be resolved by adopting the imminent quality of yielding. Try to create flexible behavior patterns and yield to sudden changes and forces that come without warning. Weather, for example, could bring your plans for a picnic to an abrupt stop. If you fight nature's flow, you meet with inner pain and struggle. Perhaps you find yourself in the middle of a verbal confrontation;

rather than force a point, win an argument or overpower another, simply yield and listen. Acknowledge the other person, validate him or her and ask that they return the favor. All conflict in life can be resolved through bending, blending and nonresistance. When you choose your battles, you usually win the war. Like the Tao, be like water and flow through the hands of those who grab at you. The *Tao Te Ching* reminds us that nothing in the world is as yielding as water.

Use the following exercises to help you cultivate persistence. Remember, also, that you will want to precede your daily workout or sports activity with a ten-minute Tao Mind breathing and visualization session to help you relax and focus on how you wish to perform your exercise regimen:

## A. BREATH WATCHING

Again, in our relaxed Tao Mind state, with eyes closed:

- Inhale slowly through nostrils and watch with your eyes closed the "white cloud" fill the lungs completely.

- Suspend breath for a few seconds (three to five) and watch the clean air travel to all extremities of your body.

- Exhale and watch the "smoky de-oxygenated cloud" exit the nostrils as carbon dioxide. See it dissolve and disappear.

- Suspend breath for a few seconds (three to five) and imagine the emptiness of your lungs.

- Repeat this breath-watching process ten or more times and notice the calm relaxation take over.

## B. VISUALIZATION

Again, in your relaxed Tao Mind state, with eyes closed:

- *Imagine* yourself becoming tired during a physical event.

- *Feel* your legs and arms being heavy and you begin to lose confidence.

- *See* the fatigue as a "friend," one who visits when you push your limits.

- *Yield* to it by telling yourself it's okay to be tired; it's natural.

- *Feel* yourself becoming energized.

- *See* your muscles becoming like water, more fluid.

- *Feel* exhilarated from finishing the event tired, yet strong and in good spirits.

## C. AFFIRMATIONS

Remember that the following are samples of affirmations that reinforce the Tao lesson to be learned. On the blank lines provided, create some affirmations that are more personal and relevant to your journey. Experiment and have fun in the process and make good use of index cards, posting your affirmations in a variety of places. Also recite them to yourself during visualization and picture what the words actually say.

When I bend and blend, I have more strength.

Without trying to resist, I can be gentle and resilient and powerful.

I have more fun going with however things flow.

Quick adaptation to unpredictable forces and change is a sign of true strength and greatness.

_____

_____

_____

## D.  APPLICATION OF ANCIENT WISDOM

Use the following pragmatic shifts in attitude to help restructure your conceptual view of the world around you:

*Water and wind are perfect examples of the art of yielding. Trust your own body to be Feng Liu adaptable. Find your pivotal center, and learn to spin from any resistance or attack. Bend to accommodate all forces, to curve around the obstacles. Get up and improvise being thrown about by forces beyond your control and begin to respond to these forces like wind and water. Dance on waves like a beachball, and sway in the wind as willow branches. Learn to withstand the weight as if you were bamboo. You are now Tai Ji dancing!*

# The Power of Modesty

Have you ever noticed that insecure people have a strong desire to promote themselves? So many of us feel the push to constantly prove our worth to ourselves and others. This need is extremely harmful to our spiritual well-being, creating inner battles and struggles that can easily be remedied with an attitude of unassuming modesty.

The *Tao Te Ching* tells us how sincere modesty invites loyal alignment with others. A posture of humility, modesty and genuine respect brings blessings from all directions. Ancient wisdom strongly encourages us to keep the jade and treasures subtly reserved within the bosom.

When you partake in athletics and fitness activities, there is always that danger of becoming very self-involved, smitten with your prowess and the condition of your body. The opportunity to display your wares, make claims and boast is enticing. According to ancient wisdom, the more you try to look good in the eyes of others, the more you separate from your heart; too much egocentric behavior ultimately creates deep-rooted conflict with self-esteem.

You begin to lose confidence, mirror the level of self-doubt and stoke the raging fires of fear, all of which create a spiritual void and a hindrance to performance. The constant need to uphold these self-centered illusions creates inhibiting anxiety and tension and a subsequent waste of energy. It seems as though the more you try to appear brilliant in anything you do, the more you inhibit the free flow of your greatness.

The perfect example of a self-involved athlete was a man from California who was nationally ranked as a marathoner in his over-forty age category. Incredibly talented, possessing all that one needed to be number one, he consistently fell short as his ego became his opponent, his ugly albatross. His bragging about his abilities and greatness, coupled with his harsh criticism of his competitors, closed off the circulation of his heart, as anxiety, tension and pressure rushed in and zapped his energy and spirit. Imagine his burden of always having to be on, to live up to and defend his ego-inflated image. The irony is, had this athlete concealed his advantages, he would not only have relaxed himself, he would have caught others off guard as he displayed his prowess, his ability to surge with incredible speed. The Tao specifically says that without action, there is advantage; don't act to be like a star and you will become one. Downplay your strength and become strong.

When you begin to experience the tendency toward self-absorption, see it as a chance to become more internally fit. Feel the lightness of being modest when you create this shift in your spiritual consciousness. For example, you can tell yourself that a modest approach will bring you inner awareness, greater success and less embarrassment over time. Being humble will bring others closer to you; they will support you. Self-illumination is a destructive pattern used by those athletes who think that promoting themselves is the way to gain recognition. Paradoxically, the humble heart is the path to honor and glory.

Being humble and low-key about your performances will also help to ward off unnecessary intimidation by others who may wish to prove you wrong, to make you look foolish in light of your boasting. For example, taunting behavior in sports such as football or basketball stirs up anger and passion in your opponents who, when the occasion presents itself, will be sure to "teach you a lesson." An excellent example of this was the championship game of the 1992 NCAA men's basketball finals between Michigan and Duke. The "Fab Five," as they were called, from the University of Michigan were seeking revenge for an early season loss at the hands of the Blue Devils. Prior to the game, they began to taunt Duke with "We're going to get you; it's payback time"—typical playground stuff. Words like these ignited a fire and Duke went on to win the national championship in a blowout, 71–51.

Learning lessons of humility and modesty will help you to become a better person in all aspects of life. According to the Tao, once again, be all that you have been given, yet act as if you have received nothing. There's no need to have others be aware of your greatness. When you really give it thought, people are uncomfortable around those who brag or boast. Have you ever noticed how unsolicited divulgence of your accomplishments, achievements or advantages tends to be somewhat offensive, turning others against you? On the other hand, if others seem curious, you shouldn't hesitate to answer their questions and give them information about yourself that could further the conversation. Look for opportunities where you can sincerely affirm yourself as well as others. You gain so much more when you relate to others in a modest way rather than being self-centered. Be encouraged to exhibit what you have been given, and willing to display genuine respect for the accomplishments and greatness of others, at all times giving them the credit they deserve. The ultimate power of modesty is not only what it can do for you physically, but the impact that it can have on your mind and spirit as well.

Use the following exercises to help you cultivate inner talent and to nurture and reinforce the power of modesty. Remember, also, that you will want to precede your daily workout or sports activity with a ten-minute Tao Mind breathing and visualization session to help you relax and focus on how you wish to perform your exercise regimen:

## A.  BREATH WATCHING

Again, in our relaxed Tao Mind state, with eyes closed:

- Inhale slowly through nostrils and watch with your eyes closed the "white cloud" fill the lungs completely.

- Suspend breath for a few seconds (three to five) and watch the clean air travel to all extremities of your body.

- Exhale and watch the "smoky de-oxygenated cloud" exit the nostrils as carbon dioxide. See it dissolve and disappear.

- Suspend breath for a few seconds (three to five) and imagine the emptiness of your lungs.

- Repeat this breath-watching process ten or more times and notice the calm relaxation take over.

## B. VISUALIZATION

Again, in your relaxed Tao Mind state, with eyes closed:

- *See* yourself in a social or group sport-exercise situation.

- *Forget*, for a moment, about how you look or what others think about you.

- *Ask* questions about their lives.

- *Encourage* them to talk about their greatness.

- *Choose* something you admire in one of these people and affirm and compliment this person.

- *Feel* the joy when you see their reaction to your giving in this way.

- *Listen* as others begin to reciprocate their caring feelings for you.

## C. AFFIRMATIONS

Remember that the following are samples of affirmations that reinforce the Tao lesson to be learned. On the blank lines provided, create some affirmations that are more personal and relevant to your journey. Experiment and have fun in the process and make good use of index cards, posting your affirmations in a variety of places. Also recite them to yourself during visualization and picture what the words actually say.

Life is so much easier when I don't have to live up to great expectations.

I see my specialness reflected in others when I see theirs first.

I have no need to inflate myself: Being who I am is already flying.

_____

_____

_____

## D. APPLICATION OF ANCIENT WISDOM

Use the following pragmatic shifts in attitude to help restructure your conceptual view of the world around you:

*Contemplate on the postures of football athletes, tennis pros, sumo wrestlers, judo and Tai Ji masters. Their true power is never obvious in their external appearances. American GIs were giants among the diminutive Okinawans during World War II. But in a drunken brawl, guess who could be the winner? Earth is the symbol of grounded modesty. Stand firm and feel modest and rooted into the ground as you practice your sport and workouts. Feel less need to boast; gain satisfaction from acknowledging proudly that you are just the way you are, a winner in whatever you wish to do.*

Y O U

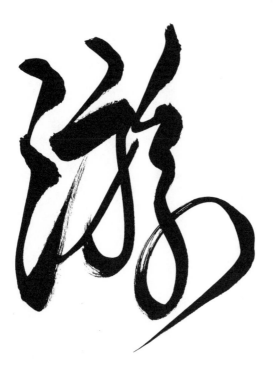

Happy wandering
Fishes in water

On this, the fifth stage of the journey, you are ready to take your inner awareness and fitness level up a notch. It is here that you will learn how to use all external movement such as walking, running, hiking, swimming, snowshoeing or any other individual athletic and aerobic activity as a means to get quiet, center your energy, reflect, meditate and silence the inner chatter and noise of your busy life in order to access your creative self. In today's fast-paced world, there seems to be no escape from beepers, pagers, voice mail, e-mail, laptops, faxes, cellulars, answering machines, and being on-line. You can't get away from all the stimulation that detracts from your ability to be in touch with your deep intuitive sense. A cyclist was riding steep hills on a mountain bike to feel the exhilaration and serene beauty of the landscape. She heard what she thought was the sound of an unfamiliar bird—beep, beep, beep. Or, so she thought! In reality, it was her bike buddy being paged by a client who wanted to ask a question that, in retrospect, could have waited. For the next fifteen minutes, she could see that he was distracted by the call, wondering how important it might be and should he cut the ride short. From her perspective, the ride was already cut short, even though they continued.

Poets, philosophers, scientists and naturalists have always known that the best ideas, thoughts and creations come to us more easily in solitude, on foot and in motion. Thoreau, Nietzsche, Plato, Einstein, Wordsworth and Lao Tzu sauntered through woods and over the hills to achieve mental clarity, "streams of consciousness," fresh original thoughts and epiphanies to help replenish their souls and sustain their imagination in order to illuminate their work and all of life.

When we begin a sports or exercise program, we do so for limited reasons. So far, on this journey, this has all changed. Our focus has gradually expanded and the global effect of our physical lives is becoming even more apparent. At this stage, you will discover how spending time alone and in motion opens the floodgates for the innundative flow of your creative juices. New ideas begin to fill your stream of consciousness as you turn inward in this state of solitude, one of the most precious assets of the physical life.

When you become silent during your physical activity, you have the chance to experience what we call "stillness in motion," a dreamy, meditative state with brief moments of quietude, as you move across the terrain. Just as a cloudy pond becomes clear when free of agitation, your mind, filled with emotional debris, gains clarity from this period of reverie or stillness within. It is a peaceful spiritual state, an inner environment where your suppressed thoughts begin to surface and visions begin to blossom, where a oneness with the beauty of nature takes place.

During this stage, we ask that you actively begin to synchronize the inner, intuitive mind with the moving body. Visualization, used throughout this book, as you know by now, is an important aspect in the creation of much satisfaction in your workouts. Combining visualization with movement enables you to become aware of the dynamic growth potential that lies within and beyond the boundaries of competition. Exercise activity offers a natural chance for short hibernation and quietude, a sense of peace and meditation, an escape from the noise of the electronic age. Like the bear who quietly enters the mountain stream, swimming around and waiting

patiently for his dinner to arrive, you to can begin to use your physical time as an opportunity to do some swimming in your own
stream of consciousness. You can utilize this meditative time to
help you to crystallize your thoughts, make decisions, solve problems, and even answer challenging, penetrating questions. This
phase of the journey encourages you to take a step back, get off the
treadmill of life and move in quiet, safe environments, alone or
with others, allowing the freshness of the day to help you find your
own sacred inspiration and personal landscape. Remember that no
one else other than you, however sagacious, can map out your own
personal existence.

In other chapters within this stage, you will become more proficient working with the cycles of change, like the moon rising and
the sun setting. "The Art of Game Sense" will help you better understand the innate intelligence of the thinking body and allow the
dancing mind to go along with what the body already knows to be
true. In the complex world of sports and exercise, with all of its
technological and scientific data, you may want to understand the
need to, as the title has it, "Keep It Simple." "Walk Your Talk"
encourages you to model, in exercise and life, the Tao of inner fitness, while "Cooperate With Natural Rhythms" discusses the spiritual act of returning to your true nature, the way you were meant
to be.

You are now ready to learn how physical exertion helps to open
up pathways to your innermost creative self and experience the
rapture of being fully alive. During this time when you work out,
when your world is free of distractions, when your mind is quiet
and all comes to a stop, take the opportunity to focus on what's
important to you and decide what you wish to do about it. It is

here that you have the chance to discover the answers to life's most important spiritual questions: Who am I? Where am I going? And with whom? And finally, the ultimate "unanswered question": What's it all about? These answers will come from the depths of your multidimensional soul.

# Stillness in Motion

As you know by now, the Tao is the Watercourse Way. Water is a universal image used by Taoists to convey lessons and truth. For example, you cannot see your image in running water, yet when it is calm, a beautifully clear, well-defined portrait appears. Developing an understanding and clarity about what is happening to you in sports, exercise and others aspects of life requires, like water, an inner stillness, in order to read and contemplate the natural rhythms and cycles of your journey, how things unfold, grow and change.

The Chinese calligraphic symbols for inner stillness represent the inner peace attained by being at ease with the receptive, open self and the calmness and clarity that are experienced when not striving.

You can achieve this calm state of peace and reflection by focusing on what we call "stillness in motion," the creation of a sense between physical movement and a meditative state. This is best illustrated by the metaphor of Taoist monks slowly walking in large circles, robes hanging practically still with each step as they meditate for extended periods of time. Because everything about us, down to the cellular level, is in constant motion it is actually more natural to meditate while moving than to sit in a lotus position for hours. You may have already noticed how movement tends to relax the body and open up pathways to your spiritual, emotional self. Aerobic exercise also stimulates a closer connection to the universe by forcing a release of natural endogenous opiates, endorphins, which create a shift in consciousness making you more receptive to deep meditative thought and overall feelings of well-being.

Stillness within is a natural by-product of your physical movement with exercise, especially walking, hiking, running, swimming, biking, skating, snowshoeing or Nordic skiing. These kinds of meditative workouts have become very popular since there's a deep need in our world for quiet, sanity and stillness, to help us reflect on the bigger game of life.

To help you to go forward with stillness in motion, begin each physical experience with a few minutes of breath watching, visualizing what you wish to do physically and carry this quiet state into your exercise. Be in the moment and tune in to your stride, pace, form, thoughts, feelings and spiritual concerns. Begin to think about your training and competitive performances. Notice what you can learn about yourself through such stillness. For example, an extremely talented athlete became despondent and discouraged by his consistently poor performance. When asked to reflect upon his life, he drew a blank. He was told by his coach to go for a run and meditate. As he started to run, he began to realize how his training had faltered because of the demands at work. He hadn't slept well in weeks due to the stress of buying a house, and he had recently recovered from a bout with a respiratory illness. In a reflective, meditative state, he realized that his performance was related to these distracting circumstances, not his athletic ability; truly, this was an epiphany.

Taking the time to contemplate the natural rhythms and cycles of life can only contribute to your inner fitness. Rather than view the beautiful flowers from the window of a speeding train, slow things down and use your physical movements as an opportunity to discover those sacred aspects of your day-to-day existence. Ask questions (the "quest" of life) that will lead you to a path of self-discovery: Why do I work out, really? What ten things that I do make me truly happy? Plan to do them each day. Try to understand what your setbacks and failures in exercise and life are telling you. How are you feeling emotionally, physically, spiritually, mentally? Why?

You need to *stop, look* (inside) *and listen* quietly to what's happening; you deserve sanctuary and time out from galloping through life. Stillness in motion helps you to grow, thrive, flourish and claim your destiny; life is a constant vigil. Your physical life is a direct line to your inner being.

Use the following exercises to help your stillness in motion. Remember, also, that you will want to precede your daily workout or sports activity with a ten-minute Tao Mind breathing and visualization session to help you relax and focus on how you wish to perform your exercise regimen:

## A. BREATH WATCHING

Again, in our relaxed Tao Mind state, with eyes closed:

- Inhale slowly through nostrils and watch with your eyes closed the "white cloud" fill the lungs completely.

- Suspend breath for a few seconds (three to five) and watch the clean air travel to all extremities of your body.

- Exhale and watch the "smoky de-oxygenated cloud" exit the nostrils as carbon dioxide. See it dissolve and disappear.

- Suspend breath for a few seconds (three to five) and imagine the emptiness of your lungs.

- Repeat this breath-watching process ten or more times and notice the calm relaxation take over.

## B. VISUALIZATION

Again, in your relaxed Tao Mind state, with eyes closed:

- *See* yourself in motion, using your exercise of choice.

- *Feel* yourself relaxed, light and gliding effortlessly.

- *Focus* on the precise aspects of your movement, the biomechanics.

- *Think*, as you move, about an important issue in your life.

- *Listen* to your inner voice as it gives you important information that you need to have.

- *Feel* yourself getting in touch with your deeper, spiritual self.


## C. AFFIRMATIONS

Remember that the following are samples of affirmations that reinforce the Tao lesson to be learned. On the blank lines provided, create some affirmations that are more personal and relevant to your journey. Experiment and have fun in the process and make good use of index cards, posting your affirmations in a variety of places. Also recite them to yourself during visualization and picture what the words actually say.

I feel the stillness inside when I move creatively outside.

My stillness sets the motion of getting rid of my commotions.

I feel calm and centered when I move in the Tai Ji Way.

_____

_____

_____

## D. APPLICATION OF ANCIENT WISDOM

Use the following pragmatic shifts in attitude to help restructure your conceptual view of the world around you:

> The Chinese symbol for gold is a perfect metaphor for inner still-ness, yet full of fire within and power in motion. Create an uplift-ing spirit with the image of a lofty cathedral ceiling above, reaching up overhead with your arms to open up the sky, to feel the light shining down into your entire body. Focus on the beam of Qi, the "thunderbolt" shooting straight down the spine. Imag-ine your crown as a rosary window to filter through rainbow spectra of light from heaven, filling every inner crevice and pore of your whole being, enlivening yourself with Qi flow. Open your arms and chest to breathe in human warmth and loving good-will. Reciprocate it by exuding outwardly your personal well-being. Now, close your eyes, sink deep into your belly to feel the FIRE of life burning. Enjoy the warmth and beauty of the flame as you settle softly into your grounding. Allow the earth below to receive and support you, providing safe sanctuary for this mo-ment of repose.

# Moonrise, Sunset

Notice the changing cycles of life. Welcome and respect these changes, says the *Tao Te Ching*. When the changes of the universe have run their course, transformations ensue. By continuing to re-cycle, they attain eternal life. According to the Tao, nothing is static; each end, a new beginning.

Nothing can be more certain on your journey into physical and internal fitness than the inevitable cycles of change. Becoming aware of and working with these natural Tao cycles create success; work against them and you upset the balance of nature. The mythological phoenix descends into ashes and quickly rises up, ex-pressing the exuberance of life. As we reach the height of our vital-ity, we begin to decline. Fire blazes, yet burns out; seas are stormy, then calm; when the sun reaches its zenith, it begins its descent toward its nadir; the moon rises, the sun sets; you win, you lose; you're up, then down; you're hot, then you're not. When anything reaches its extreme, it changes to its opposite.

Your sports and exercise performance will have its cycles too. No one can escape the periodic fluctuations of the physical life. By using the Tao lessons of reflection from the previous chapter, "Stillness in Motion," you will become more astute in predicting and understanding these natural patterns. When they show up, you will cease to fight the inevitable, become less anxious and frustrated and, by so doing, relax and profit from these swings in performance. Your acceptance of these times is a giant leap on the path of becoming internally fit.

When cycles occur in your physical program, rather than fight them, use the following Tao Mind shifts to help you feel better emotionally and spiritually: Know that the impermanence is here to stay. Ask anyone who's been involved with sports or exercise. If you do not accept this law of nature, you will experience tension, anxiety and inner turmoil. When you understand the truth about beginning and ending, you will be less likely to get down on yourself when the "downs" appear. Notice the natural cycles in your training and physical routines, plan for their arrival and adjust accordingly. For example, notice how each day you have specific cycles; first your energy is high (Yang), and then it is low (Yin), where you slow down and rest. When you become aware of your particular cycles, you will be able to successfully plan your physical activity. When you are completely fatigued in the morning, don't fight it; do your workout in the afternoon or evening.

As an athlete, you will have seasons (cycles) throughout the year. For example, if you are a triathlete, runner or cyclist, you can expect at least two peaks a year; accept this and plan to back off your training in between, rather than trying to push your way through the down period. If you plan properly, your rest periods will become times to refuel, gather your inner resources and become excited about entering the physical arena once again. All of this requires a trust in the natural process, as well as yourself.

The cycles are also prevalent in team sports; you win championships, then get dethroned. Knowing this about life helps you to accept (we're not asking that you like it) the inevitable when it comes.

Noticing these cycles in sports and exercise and then applying what you've learned to other aspects of life can save you from much anxiety and tension. Acceptance of nature's way is the essence of Tao, the Watercourse Way. You become much more spiritually fit when you flow, like the river, with the changes in your emotional landscape.

For example, you may want to honor these cycles of energy in life when it comes to being productive at work or when studying for an exam. When the cycles repeat themselves, take the necessary breaks and rest. If you break the natural law of diminishing returns, you will pay the emotional price. Rather than force your way through the work, stop and take a walk, get a snack, call a friend or do anything you can to change the energy.

Notice the cyclical patterns in other aspects of your life. Do you cook, garden, clean, recycle glass, paper and aluminum cans? Here is work of a true Zen nature when you accept the idea that things are never complete. The joy is both in the beginning and the end, only to recycle and begin once again. When you really contemplate it, all of life is one big cycle, the thought of which stimulates a spiritual quest of its own. Life is a sacred pendulum, a back-and-forth process that never ends, constantly recycling itself as it gains eternal strength.

Whether you fail, lose, mess up, succeed, triumph or perform well, feel secure in that everything always moves on and changes. Feel the joy, yet know that victory is ephemeral; experience the pain, yet realize that this setback, too, will pass. Remember that the darkest part of night is always followed by the dawn.

Use the following exercises to help you cultivate inner talent and to nurture and reinforce the ever-changing cycles of life. Remember, also, that you will want to precede your daily workout or sports activity with a ten-minute Tao Mind breathing and visualization session to help you relax and focus on how you wish to perform your exercise regimen:

## A.   BREATH   WATCHING

Again, in our relaxed Tao Mind state, with eyes closed:

- Inhale slowly through nostrils and watch with your eyes closed the "white cloud" fill the lungs completely.

- Suspend breath for a few seconds (three to five) and watch the clean air travel to all extremities of your body.

- Exhale and watch the "smoky de-oxygenated cloud" exit the nostrils as carbon dioxide. See it dissolve and disappear.

- Suspend breath for a few seconds (three to five) and imagine the emptiness of your lungs.

- Repeat this breath-watching process ten or more times and notice the calm relaxation take over.

## B. VISUALIZATION

Again, in your relaxed Tao Mind state, with eyes closed:

- *Imagine* yourself swimming in the ocean, safely near the shore.

- *Feel* yourself bobbing with the motion of the waves.

- *Enjoy* the drop from the crest of the wave as it passes by.

- *Experience* the inevitable lift from the next crest.

- *Howl* ecstatically as the gravity pulls you down, like a huge roller coaster ride.

- *Look* for some natural cycle in your life: energized then tired, for example.

- *Blend* with and accept this cycle and as you do.

- *Feel* your performance decline, yield to it and, after some rest,

- *Feel* your strength and energy come back to you.

## C. AFFIRMATIONS

Remember that the following are samples of affirmations that reinforce the Tao lesson to be learned. On the blank lines provided, create some affirmations that are more personal and relevant to your journey. Experiment and have fun in the process and make good use of index cards, posting your affirmations in a variety of places. Also recite them to yourself during visualization and picture what the words actually say.

I am ready for change when it happens.

I listen to and cooperate with nature's transformative voices.

I accept the truth of transience; what goes around comes around.

_____

_____

_____

## D. APPLICATION OF ANCIENT WISDOM

Use the following pragmatic shifts in attitude to help restructure your conceptual view of the world around you:

> I (Yee) is the classic Tao concept of the I CHING, meaning change and transformation. With the alternation of four seasons and five moving forces of nature (Fire, Water, Wood, Metal, Earth), everything is in flux. So is our energy level during our workouts. Get in touch with the inner rhythm of your body and your spirit. Entertain the changes and harness the shifting energy throughout the day, month and year. Take a few moments before each workout session to improvise on a few Tai Ji moves. As you move your arm over your head, visualize the sun rising from the east-

ern horizon to set in the west. Notice how the moon follows, appearing in the sky. Extend your vision in front and pivot all around to survey the panorama of the circle. Observe every detailed light and shade variation by shifting your perspective. Project your energy outwardly first, followed by turning inwardly. Observe and experience any change and transformation in yourself. Be thankful for being fully alive in this moment as you play your sports or exercise.

# The Art of
# Game Sense

Some of us have it, the rest of us can get it, if given the time and desire to develop it. Everyone comments how enjoyable it is to watch the young master Tiger Woods dance around the golf course, instinctively doing the right thing at the right time. Not only is he playing the game of golf; he *is* the game. He is what Zen masters call enlightened; he has the ability to see what's right there in front of him without having to analyze the situation, to do what's right without really thinking about it. According to the Samurai Warrior, his knowledge and actions are one and the same. It's called "game sense," the art of being able to see things that aren't immediately evident to most others. Game sense comes when your mind stops thinking and your body takes over, using its innate intellect. This phenomenon is referred to as the thinking body and the dancing mind. For Woods, his technical knowledge and physical prowess were only part of the reason for his record-shattering success at the prestigious PGA Masters Championship. It seemed as though he transcended techniques and power and listened to that sixth sense, the instinctual self.

The Chinese calligraphic symbols for Woods's instinctiveness describe a direct entry into the exact center of consciousness, with all instinctual senses open and focused to awaken the wisdom of inner knowing. The *Tao Te Ching* teaches that by following your heart, your instinct, you become instantly awakened, more effective and able to understand situations and react quickly and decisively. Avoid excessive thought as analysis is often paralysis.

In sports and exercise, you are given repeated opportunity to test your instinct. Rather than think about how to do it, just—*do it!* Such action requires that you let go of the need to control each movement and trust in your thinking body, its natural impulses and where they take you. It helps if you precede physical activity by being in the Tao Mind state, a place where your body, mind and spirit are aligned. For example, prior to a run down the ski slope, take five deep breaths and visualize how your body will move across the terrain, free of the usual mental chatter. See yourself dance the bumps and glide over the huge open fields of powder. Then, having done this, let your body fly as you join it for the ride. Notice the calm and ease with which you flow down the mountain when you refuse to analyze every movement.

Daily practice with your Tao Mind through visualization and relaxation will help you to see and respond to what your body tells you to do. Your best performances, those that truly stand out, usually occur when you trust and act according to your inner knowledge, the wisdom of your body, your instinct.

Through sports and exercise, you start to become comfortable with your sixth sense. Here's the opportunity to learn to grow internally by listening to and trusting what you intuitively know to be right. When you do, you invariably meet with good fortune.

You can further your development of trust in this way through careful observation of others in similar situations. After watching various athletic or exercise scenarios for hundreds of hours, you obtain a wealth of "experience" before even setting foot in the physical arena. You unintentionally program yourself to respond to a wide variety of game conditions. You develop "game sense" by watching others play, compete and work out, and begin to follow their lead. Videos such as Cybervision are readily available and are effective ways to help you develop this inner self-trust.

In the game of life, you have been unconsciously developing a sense about the natural patterns and movements, day to day. This accumulated data is real knowledge available to you through trust. When familiar situations recur, trust and respond appropriately with your instinct, knowing that not only will your action feel right, it will be right on target, according to the wisdom of the heart.

Use the following exercises to help you cultivate the art of game sense. Remember, also, to precede your daily workout or sports activity with a ten-minute Tao Mind breathing and visualization session, to help you relax and focus on how you wish to perform your exercise regimen:

## A.  BREATH WATCHING

Again, in our relaxed Tao Mind state, with eyes closed:

- Inhale slowly through nostrils and watch with your eyes closed the "white cloud" fill the lungs completely.

- Suspend breath for a few seconds (three to five) and watch the clean air travel to all extremities of your body.

- Exhale and watch the "smoky de-oxygenated cloud" exit the nostrils as carbon dioxide. See it dissolve and disappear.

- Suspend breath for a few seconds (three to five) and imagine the emptiness of your lungs.

- Repeat this breath-watching process ten or more times and notice the calm relaxation take over.


## B.  VISUALIZATION

Again, in your relaxed Tao Mind state, with eyes closed:

- *See* someone you admire in sports or physical activity.

- *Watch* this person move and perform.

- *Imitate* these movements as if they were yours.

- *Feel* exhilarated as you begin to replicate these patterns automatically.

- *See* yourself being extremely fluid and effortless.

- *Be* what you see yourself to be—You are it!


## C.  AFFIRMATIONS

Remember that the following are samples of affirmations that reinforce the Tao lesson to be learned. On the blank lines provided, create some affirmations that are more personal and relevant to your journey. Experiment and have fun in the process and make good use of index cards, posting your affirmations in a variety of places. Also recite them to yourself during visualization and picture what the words actually say.

My mind is dancing and my body is thinking.

I rise from paralysis and transcend analysis; I just do it.

I am uncluttered, open and free to play.

_____

_____

_____

## D. APPLICATION OF ANCIENT WISDOM

Use the following pragmatic shifts in attitude to help restructure your conceptual view of the world around you:

*Tai Ji dancing is the way to go! When you dance, you are not trying to get anywhere, to finish and call it a game. The game is the dance. Put on your favorite music, and boogie up a storm. Liberate your mind, heart, muscles and joints. Take flight! Learn to start fresh, untainted and like a child, enjoy the PLAY.*

# Keep It Simple

Simplicity, according to the Tao, is the great Mystical Virtue, one that touches upon every aspect of your inner being. It is often referred to by Taoists as the Great Way, the sacred, simple way of nature's most subtle law: Less is more. At this stage of your journey into mental awareness, you could be considered very wise if you decided to walk this great way, the way of inner freedom and pure simplicity. The Chinese metaphor for simplicity has one entering the bamboo gate into the open, uncluttered clearing of a courtyard to enjoy the moonlight from the sky.

The more involved you become with athletics and fitness, the greater the opportunity to complicate things. Ancient wisdom teaches us that satisfaction and fulfillment await all who keep it simple. With less to think about, there is more freedom to focus, concentrate and relax. The simple way is the more peaceful road, freeing you from the tension and anxiety of trying to complicate everything in your environment, while giving you more time to concentrate on what's deeply important. When your sport and physical workouts become so complex through the use of technology, and sophisticated gear and clothing, you run the risk of becoming spiritually empty and losing touch with the joy and your deepest, sacred reason for participating.

Take a close look at your exercise and sports agenda. Think about ways in which you can seriously create change toward a more simplified program. What's essential and what's not? Do you really need all that equipment? Will having those expensive running shoes really help you to run up that hill more quickly? If so, is it necessary to run so quickly? Do you really need to jump into your car and drive thirty minutes each day to an exercise gym when you might be able to gain the same benefits by lifting weights at home, using the travel time saved for reading or meditation? For some athletes and exercise buffs, portable heart monitors are useful and worth having, an integral aspect of their training; for others, they are superfluous gear of little value. How do you feel about this?

As you begin to feel the numerous benefits from a shift in consciousness to a more simplistic physical world, you may become motivated to do the same in other aspects of your life. Take a look at your environment, your diet, your relationships, your career, your possessions. What can you shed to create a less complicated lifestyle? By noticing this, you will begin to create much happiness in your life by following the less is more approach: a simple meal, a simple day, a simple home. There's less to worry about; it hardly matters when your no-frills ten-year-old car gets scratched in a parking lot. A computer, for some, is essential; for others, it's an expensive toy they can do without.

Creating simplicity in your complex world is not easy. It requires rethinking priorities and the willingness to empty your pockets to fill your soul. Taking a cut in salary could mean more hours with the family, quality time with your hobbies and less upheaval all around even if there's less money left over at the end of the month. It requires coming to terms with a deeper, more spiritual question: "How much is enough?" as opposed to "How much can I get?" Perhaps it means learning how to live simply in order to simply live.

Use the following exercises to help you cultivate inner talent and to nurture and reinforce simplicity in all that you do. Remember, also, that you will want to precede your daily workout or sports activity with a ten-minute Tao Mind breathing and visualization session to help you relax and focus on how you wish to perform your exercise regimen:

## A. BREATH WATCHING

Again, in our relaxed Tao Mind state, with eyes closed:

- Inhale slowly through nostrils and watch with your eyes closed the "white cloud" fill the lungs completely.

- Suspend breath for a few seconds (three to five) and watch the clean air travel to all extremities of your body.

- Exhale and watch the "smoky de-oxygenated cloud" exit the nostrils as carbon dioxide. See it dissolve and disappear.

- Suspend breath for a few seconds (three to five) and imagine the emptiness of your lungs.

- Repeat this breath-watching process ten or more times and notice the calm relaxation take over.

## B.  VISUALIZATION

Again, in your relaxed Tao Mind state, with eyes closed:

- *Imagine* when you first began to play a sport or work out.

- *Identify* the basic, simple reasons why you participated, why you love it.

- *Feel* the joy, once again, as you become reconnected with this original purpose.

- *Take* one aspect of your physical activity and experience the full pleasure.

- *Savor* it!

- *Feel* your Qi flowing throughout your body.

- *Smile* and feel yourself being free and knowing that this is the essence.

## C.  AFFIRMATIONS

Remember that the following are samples of affirmations that reinforce the Tao lesson to be learned. On the blank lines provided, create some affirmations that are more personal and relevant to your journey. Experiment and have fun in the process and make good use of index cards, posting your affirmations in a variety of places. Also recite them to yourself during visualization and picture what the words actually say.

Each day I let go of one more unnecessary clutter in my life.

I digest all my food for thoughts and keep only the essence.

I value my open clarity and have no use for accumulations.

I like being simple and free!

_____

_____

_____

## D. APPLICATION OF ANCIENT WISDOM

Use the following pragmatic shifts in attitude to help restructure your conceptual view of the world around you:

*Two Chinese symbols exemplify Tao essence: P'u and Ssu (Uncarved Block and Unbleached Silk). Before we make an artistic sculpture out of the woodblock, and dye the pure silk into rainbow spectrums, contemplate on the original natural beauty of the simple original essence of wood and silk. Before you try to impress others with your prowess and your skills in sports or workouts, return to the original appreciation of each workout's simple routine and moves. Retrace the first discovery, the joy and delight of your first attempts in executing these motions. Meditate inwardly for a few moments on the images of Uncarved Block and Unbleached Silk in yourself, before moving on to your sport or workout routines. Begin again with childlike delight and simplicity. Regain the sense of wonder.*

# Walk Your Talk

In this chapter, we ask that you consider modeling for others the lessons, truths and Tao mind-sets learned on this journey of inner awareness. By doing so, you will be instrumental in guiding others to a world that makes sense in sports, exercise and other arenas of life. With good modeling, you provide yourself and others with the opportunity to practice and solidify the lessons you have learned as you approach the "coming home" phase to your deeper inner self.

The Chinese calligraphic characters for modeling encourage you to follow in the tracks created by the wheels of a leading and guiding vehicle, much like the respect given to anyone who has paved the way before you. The Tao asks that you embrace the natural way and become the model for all. When you "walk your talk," your impact on others will be enormous and, according to the Confucian ideal, you will mirror the "superior person." If not superior, you certainly will be congruent as you display your integrity and model your Tao of inner fitness, reinforcing all that you have learned on the endless sacred journey.

In a sense, you become a sacred servant, helping others to become more spiritually rich. To use the sport of tennis as a metaphor, you "serve" the ball as an offer to begin the game, the game of inner fitness for the ultimate game of life. When another is ready to receive your service, they return it and you, in turn, receive their offering in this give-and-take dance of body, mind and spirit.

By walking your talk, you enable others not only to hear about your journey, but you make it experiential in their own lives. When you are full of postive energy, you accumulate an internal power that wants to expand to others; it can't be held back. When you share it with others, they fill their "spiritual tanks" and are now in position to have the energy returned to you, completing the circuit.

Working Out, Working Within is a journey that naturally enables you to become a teacher in service to others. To help you to walk your talk and influence others, you should create a safe, non-threatening learning environment, and encourage others to follow this way for all of life. You can do this by becoming more conscious of the implication of all your actions, words and movement. Such mindfulness, a state of relaxed consciousness, may help you to be sensitive to others and not talk about your athletic and exercise successes with those who are experiencing setbacks and failure. It can teach you to remember your own failures in times of success and can help you to instill in others their own greatness in times of their failure.

To walk your talk, exhibit the courage to be who you really are and occasionally venture into the unknown where you are not afraid to risk exposing your inevitable faults. By so doing, you will gain the loyalty of others, receive their praise and be followed by them as you act and perform out of your deepest core, your true spirit self. Welcome home and get set for a celebration in Part 3.

Use the following exercises to help you cultivate inner talent and to nurture and reinforce the concept of modeling, the ability to walk your talk. Remember, also, that you will want to precede your daily workout or sports activity with a ten-minute Tao Mind breathing and visualization session to help you relax and focus on how you wish to perform your exercise regimen:

## A.  BREATH WATCHING

Again, in our relaxed Tao Mind state, with eyes closed:

- Inhale slowly through nostrils and watch with your eyes closed the "white cloud" fill the lungs completely.

- Suspend breath for a few seconds (three to five) and watch the clean air travel to all extremities of your body.

- Exhale and watch the "smoky de-oxygenated cloud" exit the nostrils as carbon dioxide. See it dissolve and disappear.

- Suspend breath for a few seconds (three to five) and imagine the emptiness of your lungs.

- Repeat this breath-watching process ten or more times and notice the calm relaxation take over.

## B. VISUALIZATION

Again, in your relaxed Tao Mind state, with eyes closed:

- *See* yourself in a competitive situation, with yourself or with others.

- *Question* your ability and validity in this situation then,

- *Say* to yourself, "I am spiritually fit and no one can take that away.

- *See* how you walk your talk and exhibit confidence in your ability.

- *Feel* the joy as you exhibit your integrity and perform quite well.

- *Sense* the inner power from displaying your level of spiritual fitness, believing in self.

## C. AFFIRMATIONS

Remember that the following are samples of affirmations that reinforce the Tao lesson to be learned. On the blank lines provided, create some affirmations that are more personal and relevant to your journey. Experiment and have fun in the process and make good use of index cards, posting your affirmations in a variety of places. Also recite them to yourself during visualization and picture what the words actually say.

I accept the challenge of being a positive influence on others.

I like what I do with my body—a good match to my positive mind and lively spirit.

I walk my talk.

_____

_____

_____

## D. APPLICATION OF ANCIENT WISDOM

Use the following pragmatic shifts in attitude to help restructure your conceptual view of the world around you:

*Are you doing what you ask others to do while coaching them in this sport or workout routine? The Chinese metaphor of Flower-Mirror-Water-Moon is an apropos meditation. Imagine the impossibility of a deceptive mirror, flattering a wilting bouquet, or the water reflecting a full moon when it is waning. Try to match your program with what you wish and talk about for others. Take a moment to come back fully into your true sense of well-being, and affirm the coherence within.*

# Cooperate with
# Natural Rhythms

According to the Tao, when you cooperate with your natural rhythms, you discover what is right, find goodness, understand what needs to be known and create harmony in your life. Through this Tao process of inner fitness, you are better able to identify and cultivate your natural rhythms. Lao Tzu recommends that you stand strongly for what you hold to be true for you, to believe in yourself without compromise. Trust in your natural power within and use it.

On a physical plane, it is good to remember that you were born an animal. Like all good animals, you are deeply connected to a natural physical life, the way it was meant to be. By being true to this part of you, you can fulfill your own nature. Notice animals as they follow nature's way. They don't go for a workout; they don't think about it, plan it, or discuss it; they simply move naturally. They cooperate with the rhythms of nature and instinctively understand that it's quite natural to be connected to physical endeavors. As you continue your journey of inner fitness, know that the act of returning to this natural physical self, your true nature, is a divine act in and of itself.

When your natural self is rediscovered, you will joyfully return to a place where you begin to experience a free flow of natural energy. To allow this free flow of energy, be sure that you don't interfere with what's naturally happening; you need to learn to conserve energy by taking advantage of and cooperating with the natural forces of power within and without. Realize that the power of life is intrinsic, and all pervading. Harness the power, and use it. You can do this by observing how birds fly, deer run, fish swim, so effortlessly, with perfect efficiency. You need to apply these thoughts and ideas to your physical regime. For example, if you struggle to force your muscles to work, or to prove how strong you are, you will become quickly fatigued. When working out, rather than applying power or force, focus instead on the muscles being soft yet firm and imagine them working all together to make you strong. Rather than rowing your boat, try putting the sail up to catch and harness the power of the wind, a power much bigger than yourself. When you begin to feel this internally, you will begin to hurdle what you once thought were insurmountable barriers by cooperating with your more natural self.

Learn how to cooperate with your nature and try to discover the "dance" where you choreograph a sport or fitness program that complements who you are, not what you should be. It's unnatural to partake in self-criticism during this dance; create, instead, positive affirmations that nurture your natural self. This natural way encourages you to float to the top, not force your way there. Remember that your body has its own innate wisdom; know your own nature, where the tensions are and how to relieve them. Discover the "Tai Ji Boogie," which helps you to let go of all past mental blocks and barriers that impede your spontaneity to dance. Your mental controlling brake needs to be released for your physical body to move and function properly. When this happens, your natural physical path begins to broaden and expand and allows you to enjoy the pure spirit of play, the sacred magical place that has come to be known as the peak experience.

Use the following exercises to help you cultivate inner talent and to coordinate your natural rhythms. Remember, also, that you will want to precede your daily workout or sports activity with a ten-minute Tao Mind breathing and visualization session to help you relax and focus on how you wish to perform your exercise regimen:

## A.  BREATH WATCHING

Again, in our relaxed Tao Mind state, with eyes closed:

- Inhale slowly through nostrils and watch with your eyes closed the "white cloud" fill the lungs completely.

- Suspend breath for a few seconds (three to five) and watch the clean air travel to all extremities of your body.

- Exhale and watch the "smoky de-oxygenated cloud" exit the nostrils as carbon dioxide. See it dissolve and disappear.

- Suspend breath for a few seconds (three to five) and imagine the emptiness of your lungs.

- Repeat this breath-watching process ten or more times and notice the calm relaxation take over.

## B. VISUALIZATION

Again, in your relaxed Tao Mind state, with eyes closed:

- *See* yourself in your sports or exercise program.

- *Tell* yourself that you are the dancer of life.

- *Float* through your activity in effortless fashion.

- *Recapture* your innocence of childhood play.

- *Feel* free as a bird, deer, fish.

- *Embrace* your return to nature, to the animal you are.

## C. AFFIRMATIONS

Remember that the following are samples of affirmations that reinforce the Tao lesson to be learned. On the blank lines provided, create some affirmations that are more personal and relevant to your journey. Experiment and have fun in the process and make good use of index cards, posting your affirmations in a variety of places. Also recite them to yourself during visualization and picture what the words actually say.

I embody my animal power; it is my natural birthright.

I follow my nature, I am in sync with its rhythm.

I hear the music of the spheres. I am perfectly in tune.

I swim with the stream, and catch the wind and sail.

I am music. I am the dancer and the dance!

_____

_____

_____

## D. APPLICATION OF ANCIENT WISDOM

Use the following pragmatic shifts in attitude to help restructure your conceptual view of the world around you:

*Once again, put on your favorite music to dance to and be your own choreographer; provide the most natural moves for your special body and your unique idiosyncrasies. Enjoy dancing naturally just the way you are as you rediscover your own inner rhythm and flow. Be the "tiger" that you are; embrace your individual power of being. Rejoice with this self-acknowledgment and be proud of the integrity (Te) in honoring your true self. Come back to the wonderful feeling of total self-acceptance with pride and joy. Take this spirit into the next move in your sport or workout routines.*

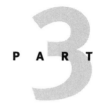

# PART 3

# Coming Home

*A Reunion of
Body, Mind
and Spirit*

You have been on the journey of inner fitness. Now it's time to come home to your familiar spirit self and notice how you have changed. You have learned many new things while gone. As you return to the mountain, it's still the same familiar mountain, but now you view it in a more sacred, dynamic way. Welcome home to your center, your heart, your core spirit where you are now at one with Tao, the way of natural truth, the way things are meant to be. Whether you find yourself in a pool, lake, river, or ocean, on a court, field, trail, or hillside, take the time to come home each day, during your solitary hour devoid of interruptions and focus on your life, a time for personal inner renewal.

In this last part, we will be contemplating the endless path of self-discovery where your inner awakening is a journey that has no destination. We will then enjoy the reunion of your physio-mental-spiritual path with a metaphor called Dancing with the Deer, a physical encounter of the spiritual kind, a mystical dance of body, mind and spirit.

# The Journey Is
# Better Than the Inn

So far, we have provided a virtual path for working out and working within to help take you beyond sports and exercise. From this point forward, we ask that you continue to travel this infinite journey of inner fitness and self-discovery on your own, using the book as a dependable, reliable companion.

What you should know about yourself is that you are a seeker; that's why you took this endless path of self-discovery. You seek the answers to life's deep, sacred questions and realize how difficult it is to discover the sacred in every day, yet this does not discourage you because there is the sense of spirituality in the quest itself. Essentially, it feels good simply to search and occasionally experience the openings, revelations and epiphanies that are an integral part of this journey. It was Cervantes who said, "The journey is better than the inn." You realize, as well, that working within is not about a finished product, something you attain as you forever sit on your sacred laurels. This book, hopefully, has "jump-started" you in the direction of the body-mind-spirit life and ignited within you the passion to continue forever.

At this point on the journey, you have returned "home," a place where all spiritual journeys lead, to your deep center, your heart; home is where your heart is, a place where your play is part of your soul, a total reflection of your true spirit. You are now ready to branch out from your comfortable, secure home base, and take numerous and frequent sojourns into the sacred land of body-mind-spirit with your physical activity, not as an act of worship or philosophical discourse, but beyond to experience the living Tao in action. Your consistent return to the Tao of Inner Fitness lifestyle will renew you and create profound feelings of tranquillity, serenity and total wellness, away from the natural mundane realities of your everyday life.

As you make your way along this never-ending path, your sacred journey without a destination, we encourage you to go beyond what we offer to you in this book. Our dream is that our work together stimulates in you an even broader perspective of sports and exercise so that you, the student, can now be the mentor helping others to be mindful in similar and more diverse ways.

Let us encourage you to see this book as a guide, not a doctrine. Its purpose has been to point your feet in the right direction. There are many paths and tributaries branching out from the main road. We know that once you begin you will create and design programs that suit your own personal needs. We want you to do this.

When talking with others about the Tao of Inner Fitness, do not cajole or proselytize; some may take offense to aligning the physical with the sacred. If you feel good about what you do; that should be enough. You cannot explain your feelings to another; one simply must experience it.

You may want to invite your children and friends to join you on a modified exercise session and use the time as a window for inner growth. The joys and inspiration experienced on a vigorous nature hike are boundless. There are many lessons to be learned by using natural events as metaphors for deep spiritual growth; respect for life, care for the earth, the cycles of nature and other sacred awarenesses as you plant the seeds of peace, love and understanding. This, then, becomes a way to bring the family closer together using what we call your spirit walk.

Remember, as well, to see the humor in all of this. For some reason, many think that inner growth is serious business, that the sacred and laughter are mutually exclusive. How unfortunate! The *Tao Te Ching* reminds us to cultivate the natural sense of joyful laughter in all that we do. It's interesting how the Tao is often referred to as the way of laughter. The Buddha awakens each day with joyful laughter, rhythm and dance. When you take yourself lightly, your soul soars. Picture yourself with arms wide open, legs kicking outward, face up the sky, laughing like the bamboo leaves in the wind; better still, do it now and see how it feels. Put on some of your favorite music, invigorating sounds of drums resonating in harmony. By doing this, you actually stimulate the release of endogenous opiates, the body's natural feel-good drug, the best medicine for a myriad of emotional and spiritual diseases. Laughter restores one's perspective and keeps the heart open for spiritual energies to rush in. Begin to see ways in which you can marinate your sacred journey in a bowl of laughter.

Let us now go forward and experience a physical encounter of the spiritual kind and let the real-life metaphor Dancing with the Deer, guide us to our own body-mind-spirit celebration.

# Dancing with the Deer

Imagine, if you will, what it would be like to integrate your body-mind-spirit as you walk (or run, or bike, or . . .) the natural path of working out in order to work within. When you do, you slowly begin to let go of the illusion of control and experience all physical workouts with a deeper, inner sense of wonder, joy and satisfaction. This can occur when you trek into the mountains, into the forest, flow with the rivers, sing with the waterfalls, in an attempt to propel your mind and spirit to new heights as you connect with the higher power, the spirit of being truly alive. A Catholic nun once claimed that she never felt more connected to her creator than she did while running through the best natural environments.

In this closing section, you will experience a magical encounter of the spiritual kind, one that can happen when you dance and play in the mountains, in the sky, in the sea, with deer, eagles, whales and dolphins, and recapture your childhood innocence and wonderment, a process of momentary bliss, a zone of calm, passionate connection to your deeper self, as two- and four-legged animals frolic together.

Here is a metaphor about truly feeling life as you embark upon an ultimate physio-spiritual experience and dance to your own inner rhythms and beats doing it your way, on your terms. You start to feel better and better about yourself and your choice to take the time to celebrate the gift of the physical life. You will begin to feel the magic of total surrender as your body becomes a temple and you cease to be spiritually homeless. No longer separated from your body, you once again become one with the rhythms of nature and somehow feel in sync with them, the way the physical is supposed to be as you coordinate body with mind and spirit. With this experience, you encounter for the first time, perhaps, the beauty of being alive and the truth about full-spectrum fitness for the ultimate game of life as you "dance with the deer."

Dancing with the deer is a real-life mystical experience that prompted this book; it is a perfect metaphor for mastering the game of athletics, exercise and life. Someone once claimed, "Exercise is boring. How can anyone exercise every day?" There is no way that one could respond to this opinion or answer this question. One simply must experience the ecstasy and joy, the carefree lightness, the tranquil calm and vulnerability that such movement and play create. For me (Jerry) "dancing" up a mountain in my Tao Mind state pricks my senses and creates an opportunity to play like a child. I try not to ponder the questions too long: Will I reach the top? Will it hurt? I focus instead on my physical experiences with the deer people, those four-legged beings who jolt me back to the primeval as they glide up the hillside doing their effortless dance over each succeeding ridge. I simply try to chase after them, hoping they will play with me. Sometimes I'm successful; sometimes I'm not.

On one occasion, I was running after a small herd when a

young buck came to a quick stop and began to charge toward me. Initially frightened by this aggressive move, I began to realize it was all in play; the deer were inviting me to join in their game; and I did as we floated together across the wide majestic mountain meadows. I was one of them; I was a deer. I became a good animal, at one with nature, in touch with a greater sense of self, feeling the magic of being in the moment and totally letting go.

As I continued my journey across more ridges, I noticed hovering above, a familiar-looking hawk who probably thought I was crazy. I knew it was a red tail by the way the late afternoon light reflected through its scarlet feathers as it glided effortlessly on an updraft. I continued to dance and flow through the steep canyons and ravines, smelling the medicinal scents given off by huge groves of eucalyptus trees. I could hear the muffled sound of thunder in the distance . . . it was subliminal. The sky to the west was a brilliant blue changing to orange and deep red. As it twisted through the atmosphere, the light from the sun created an intense clarity with all things. As the sun sets, the Steller's jays warned me that night was approaching. The moon in all its brilliance bathes the mountain in a silver sheen.

Upon another ridge at the height of dusk, I spotted a rather suspicious bobcat, a peaceful, motionless king snake and a new playful herd of deer. I wondered where they were all going—where they came from. I continued with the deer on a gallop up the next hill only to realize at that moment that I was at the very peak in almost total darkness. Obviously, reaching the top of anything is considered the pinnacle of success. At this time, however, victory for me was the joy, exhilaration, harmony and flow I experienced in the process of getting to that peak. I am a human being, not a human doing. This physical experience forced me to "be" here, in the now, during a Tai Ji run as I experienced an opening up, a vulnerability, a softness that enabled me to feel heaven from the top, earth beneath my feet, the breezes, the fire (my passion) and the water of life. I like to remain open to what runs through me, my thoughts, joys, sorrows, happiness, frustrations. I like to feel it all and, by so doing, to feel alive.

Chungliang reaffirms this metaphoric transference. Each time when he and I meet at the Esalen Institute in Big Sur, where Chungliang enjoyed many years of mentoring with mythologist Joseph Campbell, this myth-body that we live by is re-created in the mountains above the spectacular California coast highway; on each homeward journey from Big Sur to Santa Cruz, I take a moment out of the loop, stop and dance with the deer, contemplating the day's creative work and collaborative efforts with Chungliang.

Such magical encounters are available to all of us. Whether you dance with an animal or with someone you love or simply with yourself, you will recapture the physical and emotional benefits of playing like a child as you enjoy the process this dance of the spirit has to offer. Such is the essence of this Tai Ji dance, in which the physical enhances the spiritual and you begin to widen your focus as the global effects of this sacred journey become apparent.

You are now ready to take your own physio-spiritual journey, the ultimate sacred experience. Enter into your sport or physical routine with renewed enthusiasm, with a change of mind and heart as you celebrate the true meaning of exercise and movement as the pure spirit of play. Discover what awaits you when you become free of analysis, judgment, criticism and perfection, when your body becomes a sacred temple, aligned with your natural physical world.

Dive into the place of no mind, no thought, the Tao Mind, a safe, secure place of noninterference from past attitudes and behaviors. Let the earth become your canvas and nature your studio. Here it is the playful path of least resistance as you become totally natural and arrive at a place where you experience Tao. Go for it! Just do it! Feel empowered; you have within you all that you need to experience conscious fitness, to *be* physically fit in this way. Have fun and know that there really is no other purpose other than to sustain and enjoy your sport and physical activity in an effortless fashion and become more personally awakened to enjoy the dance of body, mind and spirit—the magical dance of life.

# About the Authors

JERRY LYNCH, Ph.D., is an author, international speaker, sports psychologist, coach and national-class athlete who has taught at several universities in the United States. His work in human performance has found its way to teams and individual athletes at the professional, Olympic and collegiate levels. He has written six books, including *Thinking Body, Dancing Mind* (with Chungliang Al Huang), and is the director of the TAOSPORTS Center for Excellence in Santa Cruz, California.

CHUNGLIANG AL HUANG, an internationally recognized authority on contemporary Taoism, is the founder and president of the Living Tao Foundation and director of the Lan Ting Institute in China. He is one of the most sought-after speakers in the fields of human potential, cultural diversity and creative dynamism in global business, education, and health and fitness. A Tai Ji master, brush calligrapher and performing artist, he is also the author of the bestselling classic *Embrace Tiger, Return to Mountain; Tao: The Watercourse Way* (cowritten with Alan Watts), and many other books.